Core Curriculum for Nephrology Nursing

Sixth Edition

Editor: Caroline S. Counts, MSN, RN, CNN

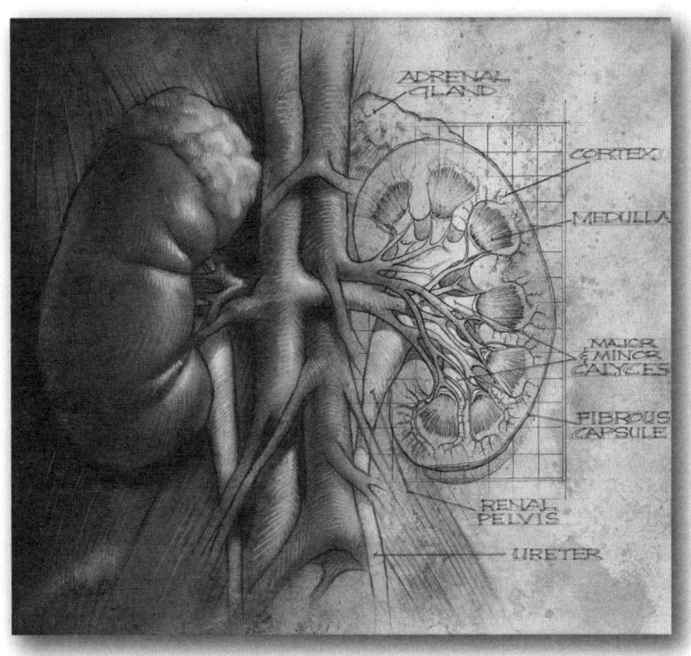

MODULE 1

Foundations for Practice in Nephrology Nursing

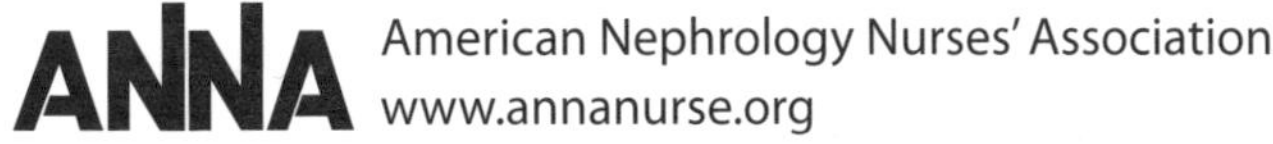
ANNA American Nephrology Nurses' Association
www.annanurse.org

Core Curriculum for Nephrology Nursing, 6th Edition

Editor and Project Director
Caroline S. Counts, MSN, RN, CNN

Module 1 • Foundations for Practice in Nephrology Nursing

Publication Management
Anthony J. Jannetti, Inc.
East Holly Avenue/Box 56
Pitman, New Jersey 08071-0056

Managing Editor: Claudia Cuddy
Editorial Coordinator: Joseph Tonzelli
Layout Design and Production: Claudia Cuddy
Layout Assistants: Kaytlyn Mroz, Katerina DeFelice, Casey Shea, Courtney Klauber
Design Consultants: Darin Peters, Jack M. Bryant
Proofreaders: Joseph Tonzelli, Evelyn Haney, Alex Grover, Nicole Ward
Cover Design: Darin Peters
Cover Illustration: Scott M. Holladay © 2006
Photography: Kim Counts and Marty Morganello (*unless otherwise credited*)

MODULE 1. Foundations for Practice in Nephrology Nursing

ISBN 978-1-940325-06-4

American Nephrology Nurses' Association, East Holly Avenue/Box 56, Pitman, New Jersey 08071-0056
www.annanurse.org ■ Email: anna@annanurse.org ■ Phone: 888-600-2662

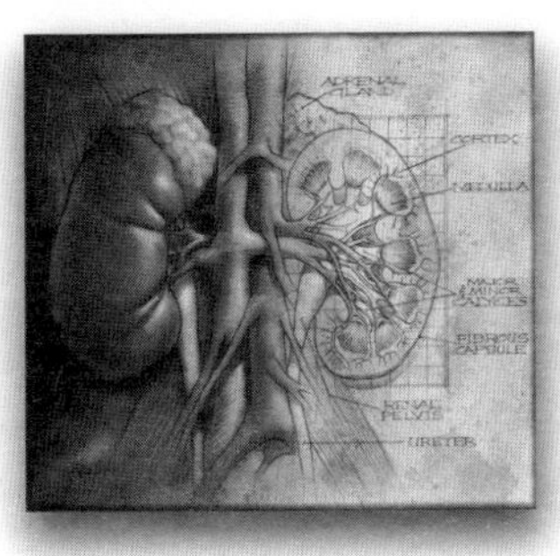

Foreword

The American Nephrology Nurses' Association has had a long-standing commitment to providing the tools and resources needed for individuals to be successful in their professional nephrology roles. With that commitment, we proudly present the sixth edition of the *Core Curriculum for Nephrology Nursing*.

This edition has a new concept and look that we hope you find valuable. Offered in six separate modules, each one will focus on a different component of our specialty and provide essential, updated, high-quality information. Since our last publication of the *Core Curriculum* in 2008, our practice has evolved, and our publication has been transformed to keep pace with those changes.

Under the expert guidance of Editor and Project Director Caroline S. Counts, MSN, RN, CNN (who was also the editor for the 2008 *Core Curriculum*!), this sixth edition continues to build on our fundamental principles and standards of practice. From the basics of each modality to our roles in advocacy, patient engagement, evidence-based practice, and more, you will find crucial information to facilitate the important work you do on a daily basis.

The ANNA Board of Directors and I extend our sincerest gratitude to Caroline and commend her for the stellar work that she and all of the section editors, authors, and reviewers have put forth in developing this new edition of the *Core Curriculum for Nephrology Nursing*. These individuals have spent many hours working to provide you with this important nephrology nursing publication. We hope you enjoy this exemplary professional resource.

Sharon Longton, BSN, RN, CNN, CCTC
ANNA President, 2014-2015

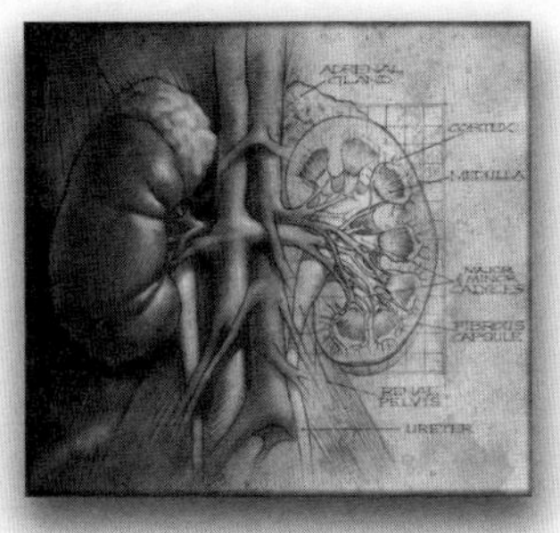

What's new in the sixth edition?

The 2015 edition of the *Core Curriculum for Nephrology Nursing* reflects several changes in format and content. These changes have been made to make life easier for the reader and to improve the scientific value of the *Core*.

1. The *Core Curriculum* is divided into six separate modules that can be purchased as a set or as individual texts. Keep in mind there is likely additional relevant information in more than one module. For example, in Module 2 there is a specific chapter for nutrition, but the topic of nutrition is also addressed in several chapters in other modules.
2. The *Core* is available in both print and electronic formats. The electronic format contains links to other websites with additional helpful information that can be reached with a simple click. With this useful feature comes a potential issue: when an organization changes its website and reroutes its links, the URLs that are provided may not connect. When at the organization's website, use their search feature to easily find your topic. The links in the *Core* were updated as of March 2015.
3. As with the last edition of the *Core*, the pictures on chapter covers depict actual nephrology staff members and patients with kidney disease. Their willingness to participate is greatly appreciated.
4. Self-assessment questions are included at the end of each module for self-testing. Completion of these exercises is not required to obtain CNE. CNE credit can be obtained by accessing the Evaluation Forms on the ANNA website.
5. References are cited in the text and listed at the end of each chapter.
6. We've provided examples of references in APA format at the beginning of each chapter, as well as on the last page of this front matter, to help the readers know how to properly format references if they use citations from the *Core*. The guesswork has been eliminated!
7. The information contained in the *Core* has been expanded, and new topics have been included. For example, there is information on leadership and management, material on caring for Veterans, more emphasis on patient and staff safety, and more.
8. Many individuals assisted in making the *Core* come to fruition; they brought with them their own experience, knowledge, and literature search. As a result, a topic can be addressed from different perspectives, which in turn gives the reader a more global view of nephrology nursing.
9. This edition employs usage of the latest terminology in nephrology patterned after the National Kidney Foundation.
10. The *Core Curriculum for Nephrology Nursing,* 6th edition contains 233 figures, 234 tables, and 29 appendices. These add valuable tools in delivering the contents of the text.

Thanks to B. Braun Medical Inc. for its grant in support of ANNA's *Core Curriculum*.

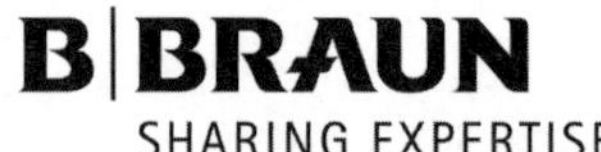

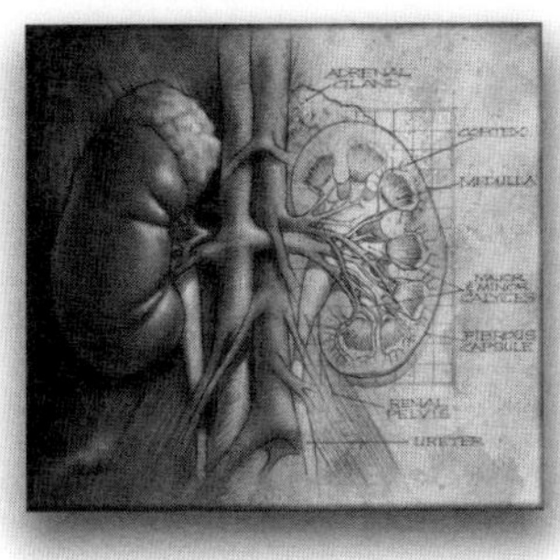

Preface

The sixth edition of the *Core Curriculum for Nephrology Nursing* has been written and published due to the efforts of many individuals. Thank you to the editors, authors, reviewers, and everyone who helped pull the *Core* together to make it the publication it became. A special thank you to Claudia Cuddy and Joe Tonzelli, who were involved from the beginning to the end — I could not have done my job without them!

The overall achievement is the result of the unselfish contributions of each and every individual team member. At times it was a daunting, challenging task, but the work is done, and all members of the "Core-team" should feel proud of the end product.

Now, the work is turned over to you — the reader and learner. I hope you learn at least half as much as I did as pieces of the *Core* were submitted, edited, and refined. Considering the changes that have taken place since the first edition of the *Core* in 1987 (322 pages!), one could say it is a whole new world! Even since the fifth edition in 2008, many changes in nephrology have transpired. This, the 2015 edition, is filled with the latest information regarding kidney disease, its treatment, and the nursing care involved.

But, buyer, beware! Evolution continues, and what is said today can be better said tomorrow. Information continues to change and did so even as the chapters were being written; yet, change reflects progress. Our collective challenge is to learn from the *Core*, be flexible, keep an open mind, and question what could be different or how nephrology nursing practice could be improved.

Nephrology nursing will always be stimulating, learning will never end, and progress will continue! So, the *Core* not only represents what we know now, but also serves as a springboard for what the learner can become and what nephrology nursing can be. A Chinese proverb says this: "Learning is like rowing upstream; not to advance is to drop back."

A final thank-you to the Core-team and a very special note of appreciation to those I love the most. (Those I love the most have also grown since the last edition!) For their love, support, and encouragement, I especially thank my husband, Henry, who thought I had retired; my son and daughter-in law, Chris and Christina, and our two amazing grandchildren, Cate and Olin; and my son-in-law, Marty Morganello, and our daughter, Kim, who provided many of the photographs used in this version of the *Core*. It has been a family project!

Last, but certainly not least, I thank the readers and learners. It is your charge to use the *Core* to grow your minds. Minds can grow as long as we live — don't drop back!

Caroline S. Counts
Editor, Sixth Edition

Module 1

Chapter 1 focuses on professional issues in nephrology nursing and is a new addition to the *Core Curriculum*. The first chapter places emphasis on nursing leadership and management. All nephrology nurses are managers and leaders, whether or not they maintain a management position. All will face ethical dilemmas; all will be involved in providing a safe clinical environment; all will take part in assessing quality care; and all are expected to perform as a professional with an understanding of what that entails.

Chapter 2 concentrates on research and evidence-based practice and what it means to nephrology nurses. It offers information on sites where valuable statistics and further information can be obtained.

Chapter 3 explains the political process and the importance for all of us to get involved. It is not as difficult as one might think.

Chapter 4 motivates the reader to prepare for emergencies. As too many of us know, emergencies and disasters do happen, and having plans in place prior to the event can help lessen the residual impact.

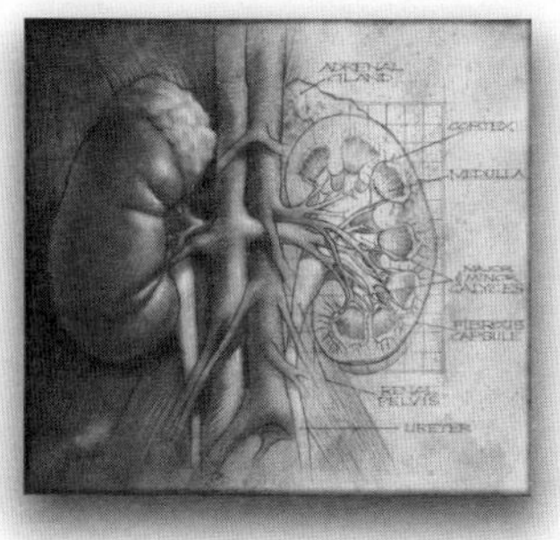

Chapter Editors and Authors

Lisa Ales, MSN, NP-C, FNP-BC, CNN
Clinical Educator, Renal
Baxter Healthcare Corporation
Deerfield, IL
Author: Module 3, Chapter 4

Kim Alleman, MS, APRN, FNP-BC, CNN-NP
Nurse Practitioner
Hartford Hospital Transplant Program
Hartford, CT
Editor: Module 6

Billie Axley, MSN, RN, CNN
Director, Innovations Group
FMS Medical Office
Franklin, TN
Author: Module 4, Chapter 3

Donna Bednarski, MSN, RN, ANP-BC, CNN, CNP
Nurse Practitioner, Dialysis Access Center
Harper University Hospital
Detroit, MI
Editor & Author: Module 1, Chapter 3
Editor & Author: Module 2, Chapter 3
Author: Module 6, Chapter 3

Brandy Begin, BSN, RN, CNN
Pediatric Dialysis Coordinator
Lucile Packard Children's Hospital at Stanford
Palo Alto, CA
Author: Module 5, Chapter 1

Deborah Brommage, MS, RDN, CSR, CDN
Program Director
National Kidney Foundation
New York, NY
Editor & Author: Module 2, Chapter 4
Editor: Module 4, Chapter 3

Deborah H. Brooks, MSN, ANP-BC, CNN, CNN-NP
Nurse Practitioner
Medical University of South Carolina
Charleston, SC
Author: Module 6, Chapter 1

Colleen M. Brown, MSN, APRN, ANP-BC
Transplant Nurse Practitioner
Hartford Hospital
Hartford, CT
Author: Module 6, Chapter 3

Loretta Jackson Brown, PhD, RN, CNN
Health Communication Specialist
Centers for Disease Control and Prevention
Atlanta, GA
Author: Module 2, Chapter 3

Molly Cahill, MSN, RN, APRN, BC, ANP-C, CNN
Nurse Practitioner
KC Kidney Consultants
Kansas City, MO
Author: Module 2, Chapter 3

Sally F. Campoy, DNP, ANP-BC, CNN-NP
Nurse Practitioner, Renal Section
Department of Veterans Affairs
Eastern Colorado Health System
Denver VA Medical Center, Denver, CO
Author: Module 6, Chapter 2

Laurie Carlson, MSN, RN
Transplant Coordinator
University of California – San Francisco Medical Center
San Francisco, CA
Author: Module 3, Chapter 1

Deb Castner, MSN, APRN, ACNP, CNN
Nurse Practitioner
Jersey Coast Nephrology & Hypertension Associates
Brick, NJ
Author: Module 2, Chapter 3
Author: Module 3, Chapter 2

Louise Clement, MS, RDN, CSR, LD
Renal Dietitian
Fresenius Medical Care
Lubbock, TX
Author: Module 2, Chapter 4

Jean Colaneri, ACNP-BC, CNN
Clinical Nurse Specialist and Nurse Practitioner, Dialysis Apheresis
Albany Medical Center Hospital, Albany, NY
Editor & Author: Module 3, Chapter 1

Ann Beemer Cotton, MS, RDN, CNSC
Clinical Dietitian Specialist in Critical Care
IV Health/Methodist Campus
Indianapolis, IN
Author: Module 2, Chapter 4
Author: Module 4, Chapter 2

Caroline S. Counts, MSN, RN, CNN
Research Coordinator, Retired
Division of Nephrology
Medical Unversity of South Carolina
Charleston, SC
Editor: Core Curriculum for Nephrology Nursing
Author: Module 1, Chapter 2
Author: Module 2, Chapter 6
Author: Module 3, Chapter 3

Helen Currier, BSN, RN, CNN, CENP
Director, Renal Services, Dialysis/Pheresis, Vascular Access/Wound, Ostomy, Continence, & Palliative Care Services
Texas Children's Hospital, Houston, TX
Author: Module 6, Chapter 5

Kim Deaver, MSN, RN, CNN
Program Manager
University of Virginia
Charlottesville, VA
Editor & Author: Module 3, Chapter 3

Anne Diroll, MA, BSN, BS, RN, CNN
Consultant
Volume Management
Rocklin, CA
Author: Module 5, Chapter 1

Daniel Diroll, MA, BSN, BS, RN
Education Coordinator
Fresenius Medical Care North America
Rocklin, CA
Author: Module 2, Chapter 3

Sheila J. Doss-McQuitty, MBA, BSN, RN, CNN, CCRA
Director, Clinical Programs and Research
Satellite Healthcare, Inc., San Jose, CA
Author: Module 2, Chapter 1

Paula Dutka, MSN, RN, CNN
Director, Education and Research
Nephrology Network
Winthrop University Hospital, Mineola, NY
Author: Module 2, Chapter 1

Andrea Easom, MA, MNSc, APRN, FNP-BC, CNN-NP
Instructor, College of Medicine
Nephrology Division
University of Arkansas for Medical Sciences
Little Rock, AR
Author: Module 6, Chapter 2

Rowena W. Elliott, PhD, RN, CNN, CNE, AGNP-C, FAAN
Associate Professor and Chairperson
Department of Advanced Practice
College of Nursing
University of Southern Mississippi
Hattiesburg, MS
Editor & Author: Module 5, Chapter 2

Susan Fallone, MS, RN, CNN
Clinical Nurse Specialist, Retired
Adult and Pediatric Dialysis
Albany Medical Center, Albany, NY
Author: Module 4, Chapter 2

Jessica J. Geer, MSN, C-PNP, CNN-NP
Pediatric Nurse Practitioner
Texas Children's Hospital, Houston, TX
Instructor, Renal Services, Dept. of Pediatrics
Baylor College of Medicine, Houston, TX
Author: Module 6, Chapter 5

Silvia German, RN, CNN
Clinical Writer, CE Coordinator
Manager, DaVita HealthCare Partners Inc.
Denver, CO
Author: Module 2, Chapter 6

Elaine Go, MSN, NP, CNN-NP
Nurse Practitioner
St. Joseph Hospital Renal Center
Orange, CA
Author: Module 6, Chapter 3

Norma Gomez, MSN, MBA, RN, CNN
Nephrology Nurse Consultant
Russellville, TN
Editor & Author: Module 1, Chapter 4

Janelle Gonyea, RDN, LD
Clinical Dietitian
Mayo Clinic
Rochester, MN
Author: Module 2, Chapter 4

Karen Greco, PhD, RN, ANP-BC, FAAN
Nurse Practitioner
Independent Contractor/Consultant
West Linn, OR
Author: Module 2, Chapter 1

Bonnie Bacon Greenspan, MBA, BSN, RN
Consultant, BBG Consulting, LLC
Alexandria, VA
Author: Module 1, Chapter 1

Cheryl L. Groenhoff, MSN, MBA, RN, CNN
Clinical Educator, Baxter Healthcare
Plantation, FL
Author: Module 2, Chapter 3
Author: Module 3, Chapter 4

Debra J. Hain, PhD, ARNP, ANP-BC, GNP-BC, FAANP
Assistant Professor/Lead AGNP Faculty
Florida Atlantic University
Christine E. Lynn College of Nursing
Boca Raton, FL
Nurse Practitioner, Cleveland Clinic Florida
Department of Nephrology, Weston, FL
Editor & Author: Module 2, Chapter 2

Lisa Hall, MSSW, LICSW
Patient Services Director
Northwest Renal Network (ESRD Network 16)
Seattle, WA
Author: Module 2, Chapter 3

Mary S. Haras, PhD, MS, MBA, APN, NP-C, CNN
Assistant Professor and Interim Associate Dean of Graduate Nursing
Saint Xavier University School of Nursing
Chicago, IL
Author: Module 2, Chapter 2

Carol Motes Headley, DNSc, ACNP-BC, RN, CNN
Nephrology Nurse Practitioner
Veterans Affairs Medical Center
Memphis, TN
Editor & Author: Module 2, Chapter 1

Mary Kay Hensley, MS, RDN, CSR
Chair/Immediate Past Chair
Renal Dietitians Dietetic Practice Group
Renal Dietitian, Retired
DaVita HealthCare Partners Inc.
Gary, IN
Author: Module 2, Chapter 4

Kerri Holloway, RN, CNN
Clinical Quality Manager
Corporate Infection Control Specialist
Fresenius Medical Services, Waltham, MA
Author: Module 2, Chapter 6

Alicia M. Horkan, MSN, RN, CNN
Assistant Director, Dialysis Services
Dialysis Center at Colquitt Regional Medical Center
Moultrie, GA
Author: Module 1, Chapter 2

Katherine Houle, MSN, APRN, CFNP, CNN-NP
Nephrology Nurse Practitioner
Marquette General Hospital
Marquette, MI
Editor: Module 6
Author: Module 6, Chapter 3

Liz Howard, RN, CNN
Director
DaVita HealthCare Partners Inc.
Oldsmar, FL
Author: Module 2, Chapter 6

Darlene Jalbert, BSN, RN, CNN
HHD Education Manager
DaVita University School of Clinical Education Wisdom Team
DaVita HealthCare Partners Inc., Denver, CO
Author: Module 3, Chapter 2

Judy Kauffman, MSN, RN, CNN
Manager, Acute Dialysis and Apheresis Unit
University of Virginia Health Systems
Charlottesville, VA
Author: Module 3, Chapter 2

Tamara Kear, PhD, RN, CNS, CNN
Assistant Professor of Nursing
Villanova University, Villanova, PA
Nephrology Nurse, Fresenius Medical Care
Philadelphia, PA
Editor & Author: Module 1, Chapter 2

Lois Kelley, MSW, LSW, ACSW, NSW-C
Master Social Worker
DaVita HealthCare Partners Inc.
Harrisonburg Dialysis
Harrisonburg, VA
Author: Module 2, Chapter 3

Pamela S. Kent, MS, RDN, CSR, LD
Patient Education Coordinator
Centers for Dialysis Care
Cleveland, OH
Author: Module 2, Chapter 4

Carol L. Kinzner, MSN, ARNP, GNP-BC, CNN-NP
Nurse Practitioner
Pacific Nephrology Associates
Tacoma, WA
Author: Module 6, Chapter 3

Kim Lambertson, MSN, RN, CNN
Clinical Educator
Baxter Healthcare
Deerfield, IL
Author: Module 3, Chapter 4

Sharon Longton, BSN, RN, CNN, CCTC
Transplant Coordinator/Educator
Harper University Hospital
Detroit, MI
Author: Module 2, Chapter 3

Maria Luongo, MSN, RN
CAPD Nurse Manager
Massachusetts General Hospital
Boston, MA
Author: Module 3, Chapter 5

Suzanne M. Mahon, DNSc, RN, AOCN, APNG
Professor, Internal Medicine
Division of Hematology/Oncology
Professor, Adult Nursing, School of Nursing
St. Louis University, St. Louis, MO
Author: Module 2, Chapter 1

Nancy McAfee, MN, RN, CNN
CNS – Pediatric Dialysis and Vascular Access
Seattle Children's Hospital
Seattle, WA
Editor & Author: Module 5, Chapter 1

Maureen P. McCarthy, MPH, RDN, CSR, LD
Assistant Professor/Transplant Dietitian
Oregon Health & Science University
Portland, OR
Author: Module 2, Chapter 4

M. Sue McManus, PhD, APRN, FNP-BC, CNN
Nephrology Nurse Practitioner
Kidney Transplant Nurse Practitioner
Richard L. Roudebush VA Medical Center
Indianapolis, IN
Author: Module 1, Chapter 2

Lisa Micklos, BSN, RN
Clinical Educator
NxStage Medical, Inc.
Los Angeles, CA
Author: Module 1, Chapter 2

Michele Mills, MS, RN, CPNP
Pediatric Nurse Practitioner
Pediatric Nephrology
University of Michigan
C.S. Mott Children's Hospital, Ann Arbor, MI
Author: Module 5, Chapter 1

Geraldine F. Morrison, BSHSA, RN
Clinical Director, Home Programs & CKD
Northwest Kidney Center
Seattle, WA
Author: Module 3, Chapter 5

Theresa Mottes, RN, CDN
Pediatric Research Nurse
Cincinnati Children's Hospital & Medical Center
Center for Acute Care Nephrology
Cincinnati, OH
Author: Module 5, Chapter 1

Linda L. Myers, BS, RN, CNN, HP
RN Administrative Coordinator, Retired
Home Dialysis Therapies
University of Virginia Health System
Charlottesville, VA
Author: Module 4, Chapter 5

Clara Neyhart, BSN, RN, CNN
Nephrology Nurse Clinician
UNC Chapel Hill
Chapel Hill, NC
Editor & Author: Module 3, Chapter 1

Mary Alice Norton, BSN, FNP-C
Senior Heart Failure/LVAD/Transplant Coordinator
Albany Medical Center Hospital
Albany, NY
Author: Module 4, Chapter 6

Jessie M. Pavlinac, MS, RDN, CSR, LD
Director, Clinical Nutrition
Oregon Health and Science University
Portland, OR
Author: Module 2, Chapter 4

Glenda M. Payne, MS, RN, CNN
Director of Clinical Services
Nephrology Clinical Solutions
Duncanville, TX
Editor & Author: Module 1, Chapter 1
Author: Module 3, Chapter 2
Author: Module 4, Chapter 4

Eileen J. Peacock, MSN, RN, CNN, CIC, CPHQ, CLNC
Infection Control and Surveillance Management Specialist
DaVita HealthCare Partners Inc.
Maple Glen, PA
Editor & Author: Module 2, Chapter 6

Mary Perrecone, MS, RN, CNN, CCRN
Clinical Manager
Fresenius Medical Care
Charleston, SC
Author: Module 4, Chapter 1

Susan A. Pfettscher, PhD, RN
California State University Bakersfield Department of Nursing, Retired
Satellite Health Care, San Jose, CA, Retired
Bakersfield, CA
Author: Module 1, Chapter 1

Nancy B. Pierce, BSN, RN, CNN
Dialysis Director
St. Peter's Hospital
Helena, MT
Author: Module 1, Chapter 1

Leonor P. Ponferrada, BSN, RN, CNN
Education Coordinator
University of Missouri School of Medicine – Columbia
Columbia, MO
Author: Module 3, Chapter 4

Lillian A. Pryor, MSN, RN, CNN
Clinical Manager
FMC Loganville, LLC
Loganville, GA
Author: Module 1, Chapter 1

Timothy Ray, DNP, CNP, CNN-NP
Nurse Practitioner
Cleveland Kidney & Hypertension Consultants
Euclid, OH
Author: Module 6, Chapter 4

Cindy Richards, BSN, RN, CNN
Transplant Coordinator
Children's of Alabama
Birmingham, AL
Author: Module 5, Chapter 1

Karen C. Robbins, MS, RN, CNN
Nephrology Nurse Consultant
Associate Editor, *Nephrology Nursing Journal*
Past President, American Nephrology Nurses' Association
West Hartford, CT
Editor: Module 3, Chapter 2

Regina Rohe, BS, RN, HP(ASCP)
Regional Vice President, Inpatient Services
Fresenius Medical Care, North America
San Francisco, CA
Author: Module 4, Chapter 8

Francine D. Salinitri, PharmD
Associate (Clinical) Professor of Pharmacy Practice
Wayne State University, Applebaum College of Pharmacy and Health Sciences, Detroit, MI
Clinical Pharmacy Specialist, Nephrology
Oakwood Hospital and Medical Center
Dearborn, MI
Author: Module 2, Chapter 5

Karen E. Schardin, BSN, RN, CNN
Clinical Director, National Accounts
NxStage Medical, Inc.
Lawrence, MA
Editor & Author: Module 3, Chapter 5

Mary Schira, PhD, RN, ACNP-BC
Associate Professor
Univ. of Texas at Arlington – College of Nursing
Arlington, TX
Author: Module 6, Chapter 1

Deidra Schmidt, PharmD
Clinical Pharmacy Specialist
Pediatric Renal Transplantation
Children's of Alabama
Birmingham, AL
Author: Module 5, Chapter 1

Joan E. Speranza-Reid, BSHM, RN, CNN
Clinic Manager
ARA/Miami Regional Dialysis Center
North Miami Beach, FL
Author: Module 3, Chapter 2

Jean Stover, RDN, CSR, LDN
Renal Dietitian
DaVita HealthCare Partners Inc.
Philadelphia, PA
Author: Module 2, Chapter 4

Charlotte Szromba, MSN, APRN, CNNe
Nurse Consultant, Retired
Department Editor, Nephrology Nursing Journal
Naperville, IL
Author: Module 2, Chapter 1

Kirsten L. Thompson, MPH, RDN, CSR
Clinical Dietitian
Seattle Children's Hospital, Seattle, WA
Author: Module 5, Chapter 1

Lucy B. Todd, MSN, ACNP-BC, CNN
Medical Science Liaison
Baxter Healthcare
Asheville, NC
Editor & Author: Module 3, Chapter 4

Susan C. Vogel, MHA, RN, CNN
Clinical Manager, National Accounts
NxStage Medical, Inc.
Los Angeles, CA
Author: Module 3, Chapter 5

Joni Walton, PhD, RN, ACNS-BC, NPc
Family Nurse Practitioner
Marias HealthCare
Shelby, MT
Author: Module 2, Chapter 1

Gail S. Wick, MHSA, BSN, RN, CNNe
Consultant
Atlanta, GA
Author: Module 1, Chapter 2

Helen F. Williams, MSN, BSN, RN, CNN
Special Projects – Acute Dialysis Team
Fresenius Medical Care
Denver, CO
Editor: Module 4
Editor & Author: Module 4, Chapter 7

Elizabeth Wilpula, PharmD, BCPS
Clinical Pharmacy Specialist
Nephrology/Transplant
Harper University Hospital, Detroit, MI
Editor & Author: Module 2, Chapter 5

Karen Wiseman, MSN, RN, CNN
Manager, Regulatory Affairs
Fresenius Medical Services
Waltham, MA
Author: Module 2, Chapter 6

Linda S. Wright, DrNP, RN, CNN, CCTC
Lead Kidney and Pancreas Transplant Coordinator
Thomas Jefferson University Hospital
Philadelphia, PA
Author: Module 1, Chapter 2

Mary M. Zorzanello, MSN, APRN
Nurse Practitioner, Section of Nephrology
Yale University School of Medicine
New Haven, CT
Author: Module 6, Chapter 3

STATEMENTS OF DISCLOSURE

Editors

Carol Motes Headley DNSc, ACNP-BC, RN, CNN, is a consultant and/or member of the Corporate Speakers Bureau for Sanofi Renal, and a member of the Advisory Board for Amgen.

Karen E. Schardin, BSN, RN, CNN, is an employee of NxStage Medical, Inc.

Lucy B. Todd, MSN, ACNP-BC, CNN, is an employee of Baxter Healthcare Corporation.

Authors

Lisa Ales, MSN, NP-C, FNP-BC, CNN, is an employee of Baxter Healthcare Corporation.

Billie Axley, MSN, RN, CNN, is an employee of Fresenius Medical Care.

Brandy Begin, BSN, RN, CNN, is a consultant for CHA-SCOPE Collaborative Faculty and has prior received financial support as an injection-training nurse for nutropin from Genentech.

Molly Cahill, MSN, RN, APRN, BC, ANP-C, CNN, is a member of the advisory board for the National Kidney Foundation and Otsuka America Pharmaceutical, Inc., and has received financial support from DaVita HealthCare Partners Inc. [Author states none of this pertains to the material present in her chapter.]

Ann Diroll, MA, BSN, BS, RN, CNN, is a previous employee of Hema Metrics LLC/ Fresenius Medical Care (through March 2013).

Sheila J. Doss-McQuitty, MBA, BSN, RN, CNN, CCRA, is a member of the consultant presenter bureau and the advisory board for Takeda Pharmaceuticals U.S.A., Inc., and Affymax, Inc.

Paula Dutka, MSN, RN, CNN, is a coordinator of Clinical Trials for the following sponsors: Amgen, Rockwell Medical Technologies, Inc.; Keryx Biopharmaceuticals, Inc.; Akebia Therapeutics; and Dynavax Technologies.

Elaine Go, MSN, NP, CNN-NP, is on the Speakers Bureau for Sanofi Renal.

Bonnie B. Greenspan, MSN, MBA, RN, has a spouse who works as a medical director of a DaVita HealthCare Partners Inc. dialysis facility.

Mary Kay Hensley, MS, RDN, CSR, is a member of the Academy of Nutrition & Dietitians Renal Practitioners advisory board.

Tamara M. Kear, PhD, RN, CNS, CNN, is a Fresenius Medical Care employee and freelance editor for Lippincott Williams & Wilkins and Elsevier publishing companies.

Kim Lambertson, MSN, RN, CNN, is an employee of Baxter Healthcare Corporation.

Regina Rhoe, BS, RN, HP(ASCP), is an employee of Fresenius Medical Care.

Francine D. Salinitri, Pharm D, received financial support from Otsuka America Pharmaceutical, Inc., through August 2013.

Susan Vogel, MHA, RN, CNN, is an employee of NxStage Medical, Inc.

Reviewers

Jacke L. Corbett, DNP, FNP-BC, CCTC, was on the Novartis Speakers Bureau in 2013.

Deborah Glidden, MSN, ARNP, BC, CNN, is a consultant or member of Corporate Speakers Bureau for Amgen, Pentec Health, and Sanofi-Aventis, and she has received financial support from Amgen.

David Grubbs, RN, CDN, Paramedic, ACLS, PALS, BCLS, TNCC, NIH, has familial relations employed by GlaxoSmithKline (GSK).

Diana Hlebovy, BSN, RN, CHN, CNN, was a clinical support specialist for Fresenius Medical Care RTG in 2013.

Kristin Larson, RN, ANP, GNP, CNN, is an employee of NxStage Medical, Inc.

All other contributors to the *Core Curriculum for Nephrology Nursing* (6th ed.) reported no actual or potential conflict of interest in relation to this continuing nursing education activity.

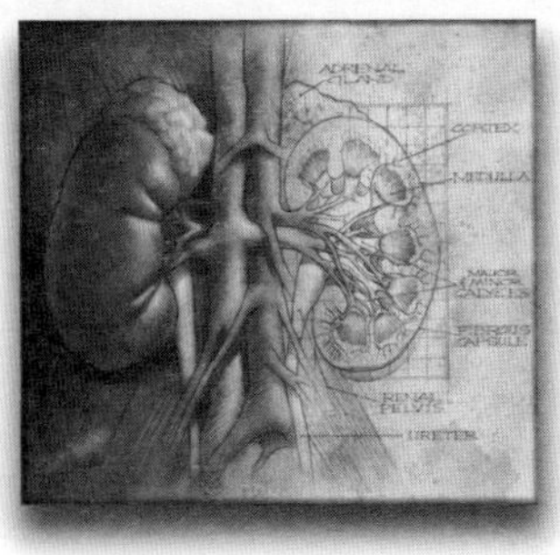

Reviewers

The Blind Review Process

The contents of the *Core Curriculum* underwent a "blind" review process by qualified individuals. One or more chapters were sent to chosen people for critical evaluation. The reviewer did not know the author's identity at the time of the review.

The work could be accepted (1) as originally submitted without revisions, (2) with minor revisons, or (3) with major revisions. The reviewers offered tremendous insight and suggestions; some even submitted additional references they thought might be useful. The results of the review were then sent back to the chapter/module editors to incorporate the suggestions and make revisions.

The reviewers will discover who the authors are now that the *Core* is published. However, while there is this published list of reviewers, no one will know who reviewed which part of the *Core*. That part of the process remains blind.

Because of the efforts of individuals listed below, value was added to the sixth edition. Their hard work is greatly appreciated.

Caroline S. Counts, Editor

Marilyn R. Bartucci, MSN, RN, ACNS-BC, CCTC
Case Manager
Kidney Foundation of Ohio
Cleveland, OH

Christina M. Beale, RN, CNN
Director, Outreach and Education
Lifeline Vascular Access
Vernon Hills, IL

Jenny Bell, BSN, RN, CNN
Clinical Transplant Coordinator
Banner Good Samaritan Transplant Center
Phoenix, AZ

M. Geraldine Biddle, RN, CNN, CPHQ
President, Nephrology Nurse Consultants
Pittsford, NY

Randee Breiterman White, MS, RN
Nurse Case Manager Nephrology
Vanderbilt University Hospital
Nashville, TN

Jerrilynn D. Burrowes, PhD, RDN, CDN
Professor and Chair
Director, Graduate Programs in Nutrition
Department of Nutrition
Long Island University (LIU) Post
Brookville, NY

Sally Burrows-Hudson, MSN, RN, CNN
Deceased 2014
Director, Nephrology Clinical Solutions
Lisle, IL

LaVonne Burrows, APRN, BC, CNN
Advanced Practice Registered Nurse
Springfield Nephrology Associates
Springfield, MO

Karen T. Burwell, BSN, RN, CNN
Acute Dialysis Nurse
DaVita HealthCare Partners Inc.
Phoenix, AZ

Laura D. Byham-Gray, PhD, RDN
Associate Professor and Director
Graduate Programs in Clinical Nutrition
Department of Nutritional Sciences
School of Health Related Professions
Rutgers University
Stratford, NJ

Theresa J. Campbell, DNP, APRN, FNP-BC
Doctor of Nursing Practice
Family Nurse Practitioner
Carolina Kidney Care
Adjunct Professor of Nursing
University of North Caroline at Pembroke
Fayetteville, NC

Monet Carnahan, BSN, RN, CDN
Renal Care Coordinator Program Manager
Fresenius Medical Care
Nashville, TN

Jacke L. Corbett, DNP, FNP-BC, CCTC
Nurse Practitioner
Kidney/Pancreas Transplant Program
University of Utah Health Care
Salt Lake City, UT

Christine Corbett, MSN, APRN, FNP-BC, CNN-NP
Nephrology Nurse Practitioner
Truman Medical Centers
Kansas City, MO

Sandra Corrigan, FNP-BC, CNN
Nurse Practitioner
California Kidney Medical Group
Thousand Oaks, CA

Maureen Craig, MSN, RN, CNN
Clinical Nurse Specialist – Nephrology
University of California Davis Medical Center
Sacramento, CA

Diane M. Derkowski, MA, RN, CNN, CCTC
Kidney Transplant Coordinator
Carolinas Medical Center
Charlotte, NC

Linda Duval, BSN, RN
Executive Director, FMQAI: ESRD Network 13
ESRD Network
Oklahoma City, OK

Damian Eker, DNP, GNP-C
ARNP, Geriatrics & Adult Health
Adult & Geriatric Health Center
Ft. Lauderdale, FL

Elizabeth Evans, DNP
Nephrology Nurse Practitioner
Renal Medicine Associates
Albuquerque, NM

Susan Fallone, MS, RN, CNN
Clinical Nurse Specialist, Retired
Adult and Pediatric Dialysis
Albany Medical Center
Albany, NY

Karen Joann Gaietto, MSN, BSN, RN, CNN
Acute Clinical Service Specialist
DaVita HealthCare Partners Inc.
Tiffin, OH

Deborah Glidden, MSN, ARNP, BC, CNN
Nurse Practitioner
Nephrology Associates of Central Florida
Orlando, FL

David Jeremiah Grubbs, RN, CDN, Paramedic, ACLS, PALS, BCLS, TNCC, NIH
Clinical Nurse Manager
Crestwood, KY

Debra J. Hain, PhD, ARNP, ANP-BC, GNP-BC, FAANP
Associate Professor/Lead Faculty AGNP Track
Florida Atlantic University
Christine E. Lynn College of Nursing
Boca Raton, FL
Nurse Practitioner, Cleveland Clinic Florida
Department of Nephrology
Weston, FL

Brenda C. Halstead, MSN, RN, AcNP, CNN
Nurse Practitioner
Mid-Atlantic Kidney Center
Richmond and Petersburg, VA

Emel Hamilton, RN, CNN
Director of Clinical Technology
Fresenius Medical Care
Waltham, MA

Mary S. Haras, PhD, MBA, APN, NP-C, CNN
Associate Dean, Graduate Nursing Programs
Saint Xavier University School of Nursing
Chicago, IL

Malinda C. Harrington, MSN, RN, FNP-BC, ANCC
Pediatric Nephrology Nurse Practitioner
Vidant Medical Center
Greenville, NC

Diana Hlebovy, BSN, RN, CHN, CNN
Nephrology Nurse Consultant
Elyria, OH

Sara K. Kennedy, BSN, RN, CNN
UAB Medicine, Kirklin Clinic
Diabetes Care Coordinator
Birmingham, AL

Nadine "Niki" Kobes, BSN, RN
Manager Staff Education/Quality
Fresenius Medical Care – Alaska JV Clinics
Anchorage, AK

Deuzimar Kulawik, MSN, RN
Director of Clinical Quality
DaVita HealthCare Partners Inc.
Westlake Village, CA

Kristin Larson, RN, ANP, GNP, CNN
Clinical Instructor
College of Nursing
Family Nurse Practitioner Program
University of North Dakota
Grand Forks, ND

Deborah Leggett, BSN, RN, CNN
Director, Acute Dialysis
Jackson Madison County General Hospital
Jackson, TN

Charla Litton, MSN, APRN, FNP-BC, CNN
Nurse Practitioner
UHG/Optum
East Texas, TX

Greg Lopez, BSN, RN, CNN
IMPAQ Business Process Manager
Fresenius Medical Care
New Orleans, LA

Terri (Theresa) Luckino, BSN, RN, CCRN
President, Acute Services
RPNT Acute Services, Inc.
Irving, TX

Alice Luehr, BA, RN, CNN
Home Therapy RN
St. Peter's Hospital
Helena, MT

Maryam W. Lyon, MSN, RN, CNN
Education Coordinator
Fresenius Medical Care
Dayton, OH

Christine Mudge, MS, RN, PNP/CNS, CNN, FAAN
Mill Valley, CA

Mary Lee Neuberger, MSN, APRN, RN, CNN
Pediatric Nephrology
University of Iowa Children's Hospital
Iowa City, IA

Jennifer Payton, MHCA, BSN, RN, CNN
Clinical Support Specialist
HealthStar CES
Goose Creek, SC

April Peters, MSN, RN, CNN
Clinical Informatics Specialist
Brookhaven Memorial Hospital Medical Center
Patchogue, NY

David J. Quan, PharmD, BCPS
Health Sciences Clinical Professor of Pharmacy
Clinical Pharmacist, Liver Transplant Services
UCSF Medical Center
San Francisco, CA

Kristi Robertson, CFNP
Nephrology Nurse Practitioner
Nephrology Associates
Columbus, MS

E. James Ryan, BSN, RN, CDN
Hemodialysis Clinical Services Coordinator
Lakeland Regional Medical Center
Lakeland, FL

June Shi, BSN, RN
Vascular Access Coordinator
Transplant Surgery
Medical University of South Carolina
Charleston, SC

Elizabeth St. John, MSN, RN, CNN
Education Coordinator, UMW Region
Fresenius Medical Care
Milwaukee, WI

Sharon Swofford, MA, RN, CNN, CCTC
Transplant Case Manager
OptumHealth
The Villages, FL

Beth Ulrich, EdD, RN, FACHE, FAAN
Senior Partner, Innovative Health Resources
Editor, *Nephrology Nursing Journal*
Pearland, TX

David F. Walz, MBA, BSN, RN, CNN
Program Director
CentraCare Kidney Program
St. Cloud, MN

Gail S. Wick, MHSA, BSN, RN, CNNe
Consultant
Atlanta, GA

Phyllis D. Wille, MS, RN, FNP-C, CNN, CNE
Nursing Faculty
Danville Area Community College
Danville, Il

Donna L. Willingham, RN, CPNP
Pediatric Nephrology Nurse Practitioner
Washington University St. Louis
St. Louis, MO

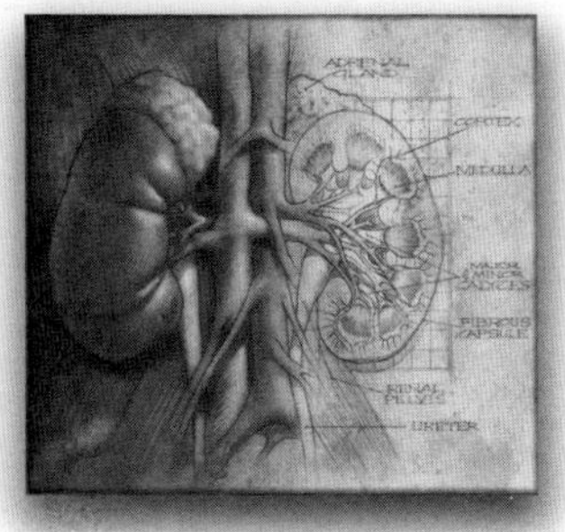

Contents at a Glance

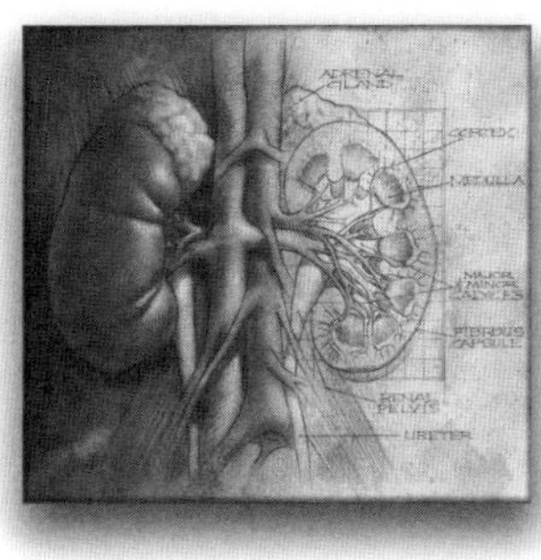

Expanded Contents

The table of contents contains chapters and sections with editors and authors for all six modules. The contents section of this specific module is highlighted in a blue background.

Module 1 Foundations for Practice in Nephrology Nursing

Module 2 Physiologic and Psychosocial Basis for Nephrology Nursing Practice

Module 3 Treatment Options for Patients with Chronic Kidney Failure

Module 4 Acute Kidney Injury

Module 5 Kidney Disease in Patient Populations Across the Life Span

Module 6 The APRN's Approaches to Care in Nephrology

Module Editors: Kim Alleman, Katherine Houle

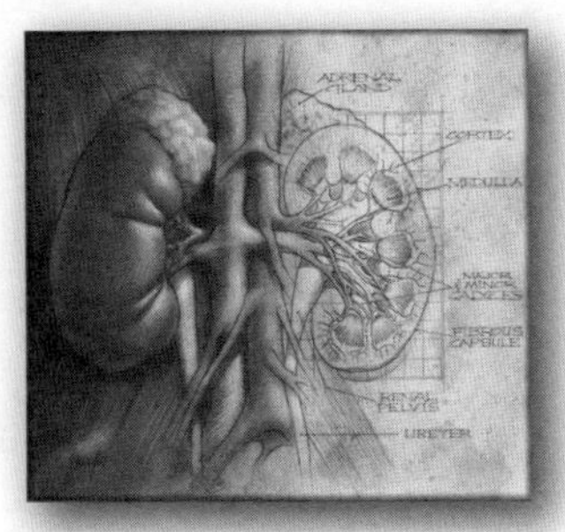

Examples of APA-formatted references

A guide for citing material from Module 1 of the *Core Curriculum for Nephrology Nursing, 6th edition.*

Module 1, Chapter 1

Example of reference for Chapter 1 in APA format. Use author of the section being cited. This example is based on Section C – Leadership and Management.

Payne, G.M., Pierce, N., & Pryor, L. (2015). Professional issues in nephrology nursing: Leadership and management. In C.S. Counts (Ed.), *Core curriculum for nephrology nursing: Module 1. Foundations for practice in nephrology nursing* (6th ed., pp.1-62). Pitman, NJ: American Nephrology Nurses' Association.

Interpreted: Section author(s). (Date). Title of chapter: Title of section. In …

For citation in text: (Payne, Pierce, & Pryor, 2015) (Use the authors of the section you are citing.)

Module 1, Chapter 2

Example of reference for Chapter 2 in APA format. Use author of the section being cited. This example is based on Section B – Standards for Care.

Micklos, L. (2015). Research and evidence-based practice in nephrology nursing: Standards for care. In C.S. Counts (Ed.), *Core curriculum for nephrology nursing: Module 1. Foundations for practice in nephrology nursing* (6th ed., pp. 63-86). Pitman, NJ: American Nephrology Nurses' Association.

Interpreted: Section author. (Date). Title of chapter: Title of section. In …

For citation in text: (Micklos, 2015) (Use the authors of the section you are citing.)

Module 1, Chapter 3

Example of reference for Chapter 3 in APA format. One author for entire chapter.

Bednarski, D. (2015). Health policy, politics, and influence in nephrology nursing. In C.S. Counts (Ed.), *Core curriculum for nephrology nursing: Module 1: Foundations for practice in nephrology nursing* (6th ed., pp. 87-108). Pitman, NJ: American Nephrology Nurses' Association.

Interpreted: Chapter author. (Date). Title of chapter. In …

For citation in text: (Bednarski, 2015)

Module 1, Chapter 4

Example of reference for Chapter 4 in APA format. One author for entire chapter.

Gomez, N. (2015). Essentials of disaster and emergency preparedness in nephrology nursing. In C.S. Counts (Ed.), *Core curriculum for nephrology nursing: Module 1. Foundations for practice in nephrology nursing* (6th ed., pp. 109-137). Pitman, NJ: American Nephrology Nurses' Association.

Interpreted: Chapter author. (Date). Title of chapter. In …

For citation in text: (Gomez, 2015)

CHAPTER 1

Professional Issues in Nephrology Nursing

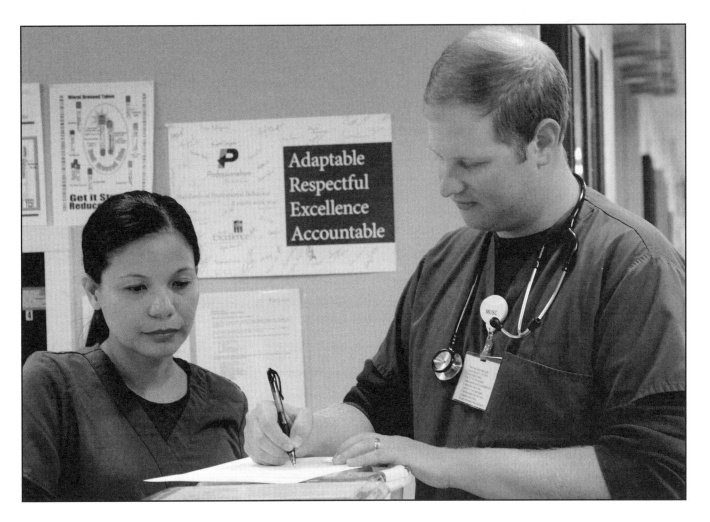

Chapter Editor
Glenda M. Payne, MS, RN, CNN

Authors
Glenda M. Payne, MS, RN, CNN
Bonnie B. Greenspan, MBA, BSN, RN
Susan A. Pfettscher, PhD, RN
Nancy B. Pierce, BSN, RN, CNN
Lillian A. Pryor, MSN, RN, CNN

CHAPTER 1
Professional Issues in Nephrology Nursing

This offering for **1.4 contact hours** is provided by the American Nephrology Nurses' Association (ANNA).

American Nephrology Nurses' Association is accredited as a provider of continuing nursing education by the American Nurses Credentialing Center Commission on Accreditation.

ANNA is a provider approved by the California Board of Registered Nursing, provider number CEP 00910.

This CNE offering meets the continuing nursing education requirements for certification and recertification by the Nephrology Nursing Certification Commission (NNCC).

To be awarded contact hours for this activity, read this chapter in its entirety. Then complete the CNE evaluation found at **www.annanurse.org/corecne** and submit it; or print it, complete it, and mail it in. Contact hours are not awarded until the evaluation for the activity is complete.

Example of reference in APA format. Use author of the section being cited. This example is based on Section C – Leadership and Management.

Payne, G.M., Pierce, N., & Pryor, L. (2015). Professional issues in nephrology nursing: Leadership and management. In C.S. Counts (Ed.), *Core curriculum for nephrology nursing: Module 1. Foundations for practice in nephrology nursing* (6th ed., pp. 1-62). Pitman, NJ: American Nephrology Nurses' Association.

Interpreted: Section author(s). (Date). Title of chapter: Title of section. In …

Cover photo by Counts/Morganello.

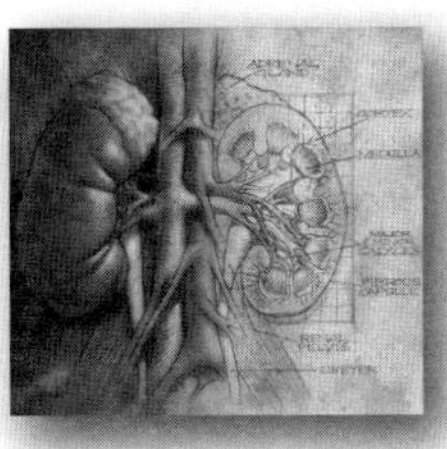

CHAPTER 1

Professional Issues in Nephrology Nursing

Purpose

This chapter provides a broad overview of important issues that challenge nephrology nurses in their work places, with sufficient detail to allow for understanding and growth as a professional.

Objectives

Upon completion of this chapter, the learner will be able to:

1. Describe the nephrology nurse's role in the broader healthcare environment.
2. Discuss principles of ethics and ethical dilemmas in the care of individuals with kidney disease.
3. Recognize effective leadership and management decisions.
4. Identify key components of a quality assessment and performance improvement (QAPI) program.
5. Describe the role of accreditation organizations and regulatory agencies at the state and federal levels.

SECTION A
Professional Issues

Glenda M. Payne

I. Introduction.

A. *Merriam-Webster's Online Dictionary* (n.d.) defines professionalism as "the skill, good judgment, and polite behavior that is expected from a person who is trained to do a job well."

B. The National Labor Relations Board, through the National Labor Relations Act (NRLA), includes the following in their definition of professional employees:
  1. Predominantly intellectual and varied in character as opposed to routine mental, manual, mechanical, or physical work.
  2. Involving the consistent exercise of discretion and judgment in its performance.
  3. Of such character that the output produced or the result accomplished cannot be standardized in relation to a given period of time.
  4. Requiring knowledge of an advanced type in a field of science or learning customarily acquired by a prolonged course of specialized intellectual instruction and study in an institution of higher learning or a hospital, as distinguished from a general academic education or from an apprenticeship, or training in the performance of routine mental, manual, or physical processes (National Labor Relations Act, 1935).

C. Nephrology nurses are trained to do many jobs well.
  1. With new opportunities opening daily, nephrology nurses may choose to practice in chronic kidney disease (CKD) clinics, transplant programs, hospital nephrology units, pediatric dialysis or transplant programs, home therapy programs, outpatient or acute dialysis facilities, informatics, academia, government agencies, corporate programs in biotechnology, pharmacology or organization management, or research.
  2. Nephrology nurses may provide direct clinical care, management, leadership, education, or research.

D. Whatever the practice setting and services provided, the rate of change in our healthcare delivery systems makes it increasingly difficult to maintain the skill and judgment (which must be based on up-to-date knowledge) critical to the professional practice of nursing.

E. This chapter provides basic information critical for every nephrology nurse. As professionals, nurses engage in work that is predominantly intellectual and varied dependent upon the nature of the work and the practice setting. Nurses use consistent discretion and judgment in their practice, require knowledge of an advanced type, and engage in continuous learning throughout their professional career (Styles, 1982).

II. ANNA *Nephrology Nursing Scope and Standards of Practice* (Gomez, 2011). First published in 1977, and most recently revised in 2011, this text defines the standards of clinical practice and professional performance for all nephrology nurses in the provision of high-quality care for individuals with kidney disease. Nephrology nurses should put the scope and standards into operation and share them with the interdisciplinary team in an effort to standardize care.

A. The standards of nephrology nursing practice are authoritative statements of the duties that all nephrology registered nurses are expected to perform competently.

B. The scope and standards provide nephrology nurses with a process for not only defining the scope of practice, but also a way to evaluate that practice. Standards can be used:
   1. To implement quality improvement.
   2. To develop policies, procedures, position descriptions, performance appraisals, educational programs, patient education, and outcome evaluation tools.
   3. In research.

C. The standards may serve to gauge the quality of care provided to patients with the understanding that the application of the standards is context dependent. The standards are "subject to change with the dynamics of the nursing profession, nephrology practice, and local, state and federal regulation. In addition, specific conditions and clinical circumstances may affect the application of the standards at a given time, e.g., during a natural disaster" (Gomez, 2011, p. 15).

D. The 7th edition of ANNA's *Nephrology Nursing Scope and Standards of Practice* is based on *Nursing: Scope and Standards of Practice,* published by the American Nurses Association (ANA) (2010).
   1. These standards include competencies rather than measurement criteria. Competency is defined as "an expected level of performance that integrates knowledge, skills, abilities, and judgment" (Gomez, 2011, p. 15).
   2. Both ANA and ANNA incorporate the advanced practice registered nurse (APRN) into their overall standards.

E. Definition of nephrology nursing. "Nephrology nursing is a specialty practice addressing the protection, promotion, and optimization of the health and well-being of individuals with kidney disease. These goals are achieved through the prevention and treatment of illness and injury, and the alleviation of suffering through patient, family, and community advocacy" (Gomez, 2011, p. 1).

F. Scope of practice for nephrology nursing. "Nephrology nursing encompasses the primary, secondary, and tertiary care of individuals with potential and progressive chronic kidney disease, end-stage renal disease, acute kidney injury, and other healthcare conditions requiring nephrologic intervention. Nephrology nursing practice spans the continuum of care for patients with kidney disease. Nephrology nurses provide care to neonatal, pediatric, adult, and geriatric individuals from a variety of ethnic groups" (Gomez, 2011, p 1).

G. ANNA's Standards of Nephrology Nursing Practice describe competencies in the following areas:
   1. Assessment: collecting comprehensive data pertinent to the healthcare consumer's health and/or the situation (p. 16).
   2. Diagnosis: analyzing the assessment data to determine the diagnoses or the issues (p. 18).
   3. Outcomes identification: identifying expected outcomes for a plan individualized to the healthcare consumer or the situation (p. 19).
   4. Planning: developing a plan that prescribes strategies and alternatives to attain expected outcomes (p. 20).
   5. Implementation: implementing the identified plan (p. 21).
      a. Coordination of care delivery.
      b. Health teaching and health promotion to promote health and a safe environment (p. 23).
      c. Consultation: to influence the identified plan, enhance the abilities of others, and effect change (p. 24).
      d. Prescriptive authority and treatment: the APRN uses prescriptive authority, procedures, referrals, treatment, and therapies in accordance with state and federal laws and regulations (p. 24).
   6. Evaluation: evaluating progress toward attainment of outcomes (p. 25).

H. The nephrology nursing Standards of Professional Performance describe competencies for the following areas:
   1. Ethics: nephrology registered nurses practice ethically (p. 27).
   2. Education: nephrology registered nurses attain knowledge and competence that reflect current nursing practice (p. 28).

3. Evidence-Based Practice and Research: nephrology registered nurses integrate evidence and research findings into practice (p. 29).
4. Quality of Practice: nephrology registered nurses contribute to quality nursing practice (p. 30).
5. Communication: nephrology registered nurses communicate effectively in a variety of formats in all areas of practice (p. 31).
6. Leadership: nephrology registered nurses demonstrate leadership in the professional practice setting and the profession (p. 32).
7. Collaboration: nephrology registered nurses collaborate with the healthcare consumer, family, and others in the conduct of nephrology nursing practice (p. 33).
8. Professional Practice Evaluation: nephrology registered nurses evaluate her/his own practices in relation to professional practice standards and applicable guidelines, statutes, rules, and regulations (p. 34).
9. Resource Utilization: nephrology registered nurses use appropriate resources in a way that is safe, effective, and financially responsible (p. 35).
10. Environmental Health: nephrology registered nurses practice in an environmentally safe and healthy manner (p. 36).

I. The standards are subject to formal, periodic review and revision. See the Standard section on evidence-based practice in Chapter 2 of this module for a historical overview of the development of the ANNA Scope and Standards.

III. The American Nurses Association (ANA) connection.

ANNA is an organizational affiliate of the ANA. This means ANNA leaders attend and participate in national ANA meetings and routinely receive correspondence, as well as opportunities for member participation, to ensure the voices of nephrology nurses are included when ANA "speaks" for nursing. In the changing healthcare environment, it is critical that the voice of nursing is clearly an equal part of the conversations that shape the care delivery systems of the future.

A. In 2005, ANNA submitted an application to ANA's Congress of Nursing Practice and Economics (the Congress) to seek recognition as a nursing specialty.
   1. After reviewing the application, the Congress found all criteria had been met for the designation of nephrology nursing as a recognized nursing specialty.
   2. In addition, the Congress approved the published nephrology nursing scope of practice statement and acknowledged the published nephrology nursing standards of practice.
   3. ANA provides these services to the nursing profession because of the rapidly changing healthcare environment. The Association has in place a consistent, standardized process for recognizing specialty areas of nursing practice, approving scope of practice statements, and acknowledging specialty nursing standards.

B. ANA's *Nursing: Scope and Standards of Practice* describes the art and science of nursing (ANA, 2010a), and was used as a blueprint when ANNA developed the *Nephrology Nursing Scope and Standards of Practice.*

C. As the "umbrella" organization encompassing all nurses, ANA serves as the national spokesperson for nursing. In 2014, ANA's advocacy programs focused on:
   1. Safe staffing. ANA is supporting state and federal legislation to require hospitals to develop and implement nurse staffing plans that are developed by direct care registered nurses, based on each unit's unique circumstances and changing needs.
   2. Reducing limits on practice for APRNs. ANA is supporting a change in the federal laws to allow APRNs to sign home health plans of care and certify Medicare patients for the home health benefit.
   3. Safe patient handling and mobility (SPHM). ANA advocates for recognition of the impact of staff injuries from manual lifting and transfers of patients, and for policies that result in the elimination of manual lifting. Part of this advocacy is in the support and publication of research to demonstrate that a successful SPHM program can increase patient safety and decrease staff injuries, while increasing nurse retention, recruitment, and retention (ANA 2014).
   4. Proposed changes in the Veteran's Hospital Administration (VHA) Nursing Handbook that would recognize APRNs as independent practitioners throughout the VHA system. ANA is supporting these changes as they would remove artificial barriers, increase access to healthcare services, reduce costs, and improve the quality of health care provided to veterans. The proposed change would allow APRNs to practice to the full capacity of their education and clinical expertise, without regard to the idiosyncrasies of state laws. This change is congruent with the 2010 recommendations from the Institute of Medicine (see the following information).

IV. Institute of Medicine (IOM) Report on the Future of Nursing (FON) (2011).

A. The committee responsible for the IOM FON report included experts in public health, medicine, pharmacology, business, and academia as well as nursing leaders.

B. The Report recognizes the critical importance of well-educated registered nurses in the changing healthcare environment as access to care is increased by provisions of the Affordable Care Act (ACA). These were the key recommendations of this IOM report (p. 4):
   1. Nurses should practice to the full extent of their education and training.
   2. Nurses should achieve higher levels of education and training through an improved education system that promotes seamless academic progression. (The FON report recommended that by 2020, 80% of registered nurses should be BSN-prepared and the number of doctorate prepared nurses should be doubled.)
   3. Nurses should be full partners with physicians and other healthcare professionals in redesigning healthcare in the United States.
   4. Effective workforce planning and policy making require better data collection and information infrastructure.

C. What the IOM FON report means for ANNA. To meet the recommendations of this IOM report, ANNA:
   1. Designs educational programs to enhance the knowledge and skills of nephrology nurses.
   2. Provides scholarships and grants in support of education and research.
   3. Actively collaborates with other nephrology professional organizations to demonstrate the value of nursing and advocates for nurses to practice as full partners with physicians.
   4. Surveys and educates members on workforce planning and the construction of a more robust data infrastructure.

V. Licensure. Each nurse is responsible to his/her state's Board of Nursing.

A. Nurse Practice Acts (NPA). Each state requires a nurse to be licensed to practice nursing in that state. The NPA may "stand alone" or be combined with licensing requirements for other healthcare professionals. Each nurse is responsible for knowing and understanding the NPA in the state(s) in which he or she practices.
   1. Rules related to delegation. Many NPAs include or reference limits on practices that may be delegated.
      a. Most states, if not all, prohibit the delegation of patient assessment.
      b. Many states limit delegation of medication administration, which can prohibit administration of heparin by a patient care technician (PCT) as a part of a routine hemodialysis treatment.
      c. Some states limit care of central venous catheters (to include initiation and termination of hemodialysis treatment and exit site care) to registered nurses.
   2. O'Keefe (2014), in an article in the *Nephrology Nursing Journal,* provided a guide to the limits various states place on clinical tasks that may be delegated by RNs to LPNs/LVNs and PCTs.

B. Nurse Licensure Compact (NLC). The NLC is a method to extend a license to practice as a registered nurse from the state where the nurse resides to all the states that participate in the NLC.
   1. Nurses whose practices include provision of service to a patient in another state, which is common in case management and in telehealth, are expected to be licensed in the state where the patient is located at the time of service. The NLC allows practice across state lines when both states participate in the Compact.
   2. Emergency staffing following a disaster, such as a hurricane or a winter storm, is greatly facilitated when the states needing help and the states sending help both participate in the NLC.
   3. Nurses who practice in states that participate in the Compact are expected to know and follow the NPA of each of the states in which they practice.
   4. Each state must pass a law to adopt the NLC. At the time of publication, 24 states were members of the Compact. For more information and a current list of member states, go to https://www.ncsbn.org/nlc.htm

VI. Certification. Individual certification is one means of demonstrating commitment to high-quality practice.

A. ANNA supports certification as "an essential component to the internal management of specialty nursing practice" and believes that certification "assists in protecting the public from unsafe and incompetent caregivers" (ANNA, 2013).

B. Certification bodies require:
   1. Varying levels of experience to qualify to take their exams.
   2. Documentation of continuing education to maintain certification. See their websites (listed below) for up-to-date information.

C. Some employers require certification for specific positions, such as facility or regional educators. Some employers include certification as a requirement in their clinical ladder.

D. Certification fulfills a personal desire to demonstrate a level of expertise in one's chosen specialty.

E. Certification agencies for nephrology nurses include:
   1. The Nephrology Nursing Certification Commission (NNCC), an independent credentialing organization that offers the following certifications for nephrology nurses:
      a. Certified Dialysis Licensed Practical Nurse / Licensed Vocational Nurse (CD-LPN/LVN).
      b. Certified Dialysis Nurse (CDN).
      c. Certified Nephrology Nurse (CNN).
      d. Certified Nephrology Nurse – Nurse Practitioner (CNN-NP).
      e. For more information, visit http://www.nncc-exam.org
   2. The American Board for Transplant Certification (ABCT) is an independent credentialing organization that offers certification for transplant professionals to include:
      a. Certified Procurement Transplant Coordinator (CPTC).
      b. Certified Clinical Transplant Coordinator (CCTC).
      c. Certified Clinical Transplant Nurse (CCTN).
      d. For more information,visit http://www.natco1.org/Professional-Development/ABTC.asp
   3. The Board of Nephrology Examiners for Nurses and Technicians (BONENT) is a nonprofit, independent certification organization that offers the following certifications for nephrology nurses:
      a. Certified Hemodialysis Nurse (CHN).
      b. Certified Peritoneal Dialysis Nurse (CPDN).
      c. For more information: http://www.bonent.org

SECTION B

Ethics

Susan A. Pfettscher

I. Bioethics: definition and history.

A. Branch of philosophy – moral philosophy.

B. Attempts to define the right and wrong behaviors of individuals, groups, and societies based on multiple defined principles.
   1. Shared agreement among people or groups.
   2. If shared by the majority, an ethical belief may become law in a state and/or country. Example: nondiscrimination based on age, gender, or race/ethnicity.
   3. If beliefs are not shared by a vast majority, they remain controversial for individuals and groups and may not be made law, although some become law and remain controversial. Individual/group beliefs may be based on other sets of beliefs (e.g., religious, societal, organizational, or institutional).

C. Moral beliefs and behaviors based on those beliefs may or may not be universal; all societies throughout the world may not share or define the beliefs in the same way.

D. Origins of (bio)ethics found in Greek philosophy (Jonsen, 1998).
   1. Greek philosophers established rules for the behavior of the Greek citizens.
   2. Hippocrates, the Greek physician-philosopher, provided the first ethical principle of medicine in his statement, "First, do no harm," and other less well-known beliefs.
      a. Became the basic tenet of Western medicine over the course of its development.
      b. Expressed in the Hippocratic Oath, taken by graduating physicians in many medical schools.
   3. Judaic beliefs expressed in the Ten Commandments.
      a. "Thou shalt not kill" applied to medicine.
      b. Extends to a belief that suicide is wrong.

E. Christian religious beliefs shared the Ten Commandments and added the Christian belief of "Do unto others as they would do unto you," incorporating the idea of intentionally not only doing no harm, but also of doing good.
   1. Became the underlying principle for taking care of other persons in their time of need.
   2. Expressed by nuns and priests in the development of hospices and hospitals over the centuries to provide medical care.

F. Judeo-Christian principles, and principles promulgated by modern philosophers, are all used in defining the ethical practice of health care and in the resolution of ethical dilemmas.

G. Eastern cultures and societies have similarly developed principles of behavior that are applied to healthcare practices (e.g., beliefs about death and dying, decision making, autonomy, donation of organs and tissues).

II. Review of ethics principles (Husted & Husted, 2008; Jonsen et al., 2006; Lachman, 2006).

A. Patients with CKD in stages 2, 3, 4 receive treatments that are qualitatively and quantitatively different from the treatments of patients with CKD stage 5, i.e., dialysis and transplantation.

1. While advanced practice registered nurses (APRNs) may be caring for these patients and may be confronting some ethical dilemmas in their care, the majority of nephrology nurses do not establish a relationship with the patient with CKD until he or she is beginning kidney replacement therapy (KRT).
2. Nephrology nurses who perform a specific task such as options education may identify an ethical dilemma or conflict for the patient, and should take action(s) (described below) to resolve the problem.
3. The ethics principles that may play a role in the patient's decision making or choices may change as the patient progresses through the stages of chronic kidney disease.
4. In addition, many patients with CKD who remain in stages 2, 3, or 4 may not ever have to make decisions about the use of replacement therapy (dialysis and/or transplantation) to treat their illness.

B. General ethics principles, as identified and written about by philosophers, have been applied to health care in the modern era.
  1. *Beneficence:* act of doing good.
    a. Application to health care.
      (1) Practitioners and others affiliated with health care in the United States generally believe they are doing good for the recipients of health care (and their loved ones) and that actions taken will result in recovery from illness or disease or improvement in health status.
      (2) While actions may cause pain or distress in reaching this outcome, these negative events are usually momentary, short-term, and/or can be relieved in some way.
    b. Results.
      (1) Healthcare interventions are good.
      (2) The people who work in health care are good, well-meaning people.
      (3) Their beneficiaries have improvement in their lives from the interventions of the healthcare providers.
    c. Application to the treatment of CKD.
      (1) Presumes that death is the enemy, is bad, and that no one wants to die.
      (2) Thus, dialysis or transplant as life-saving treatments are good (Russ et al., 2005, 2007).
    d. Question for reflection: Does everyone agree what constitutes beneficence for the entire population, for a group of people, for other individuals, for loved ones, or for oneself?
  2. *Nonmaleficence*: modern interpretation of doing no harm.
    a. Often considered the opposite of beneficence but may not be.
    b. By doing no harm:
      (1) We may not be doing anything beneficial in a positive way.
      (2) May only be maintaining the status quo and allowing health status deterioration until death occurs.
    c. Application to treatment of CKD stages 1 to 5.
      (1) Not initiating treatment if the recipient believes that it would cause greater harm.
      (2) Maintaining central venous catheters when there are no identifiable sites for creating an internal access (do no harm = protect the patient from possible complications caused by unsuccessful surgery).
  3. *Futility*: nothing more can be provided in a beneficent and/or nonmaleficent way (Rinehart, 2013; Rivin, 1997).
    a. A modern acknowledgment that technologies and interventions are maintaining biologic life without any chance of improvement in the patient's health status. This term is often applied to patients who are comatose, in vegetative states, or who have no other treatment options (e.g., patients with end-stage cancer for whom no further treatment is available).
    b. Provides an opportunity for the healthcare team to offer and provide palliative, end-of-life, or hospice care.
    c. Futility is incompatible with a belief in miracles or a belief that one should not discontinue treatment (e.g., belief that only God or a higher power can decide when life should end).
    d. Application to treatment of CKD stages 1 to 5.
      (1) May be used as a rationale for a patient's decision to discontinue dialysis (life is not worth living).
      (2) When legal surrogates are asked to make decisions regarding discontinuation of treatment when the patient is unable to express his/her wishes (e.g., due to stroke, septicemia with neurologic injury). On the contrary, if patients and/or surrogates do not believe in futility, they will not allow dialysis to be discontinued.
      (3) For a patient with a failing kidney transplant, discussions of the need to return to dialysis may be complicated by the patient's inability to believe or acknowledge that the transplanted kidney has failed.
    e. Healthcare professionals may also have different beliefs regarding the principle of futility. Expressions such as *fighting disease*, *being courageous*, or *never giving up* may

suggest that the professional does not believe in the principle of futility and may not support discontinuation of treatment.

4. *Autonomy*: the right of the individual (patient) to make any and all decisions about his/her life.
   a. Considered a right of adulthood in Western societies but is not a universally shared principle.
   b. Provides the right of an individual to make all decisions about his/her health care and treatments. Autonomy is codified in legislation including Informed Consent for Treatment, Advance Directives, or Durable Power of Attorney.
   c. Ensures that no one can provide medical treatments to a person without his/her consent.
   d. Adults are encouraged to record their wishes about health care and treatment, but there is no legal requirement for this.
   e. Application to treatment of CKD stages 1 to 5.
      (1) The professional staff members are mandated to inform, educate, and support patients in exercising their right to complete an Advance Directive. More information on end-of-life care is provided in Module 2 of the *Core Curriculum*.
      (2) Patients sign informed consents for dialysis treatment, administration of certain drugs and vaccines, and reuse of dialyzers; the staff is obligated to ensure that the patient understands what he/she is signing and is competent to sign.
      (3) As in other health facilities, dialysis clinic staff are required to adhere to patients' wishes when expressed in an Advance Directive or any other form (e.g., Physician Orders for Life Sustaining Treatment (POLST), Medical Orders for Life Sustaining Treatment [MOLST], handwritten document) used by an individual to express his/her wishes.
      (4) Staff can and should provide information about an Advance Directive but cannot be involved in the completion of documents (should not serve as a witness or named agent).
      (5) Completion of an Advance Directive, POLST, or MOLST allows the patient to continue or discontinue CKD stage 5 treatment whenever he/she wants irrespective of the wishes or interference by family, significant others, or healthcare professionals (Moss, 2011).
      (6) While an Advance Directive is most frequently written to express wishes regarding initiation or discontinuation of treatment, it can also serve to indicate how long treatment should continue and what types of treatments a patient does wish to receive.
      (7) Advance Directive/Durable Power of Attorney for Health Care documents are also completed to ask another person to make decisions on behalf of an individual.
         (a) Such a document is especially useful if the parties have had discussions about the wishes to be carried out.
         (b) If a surrogate does not know what the patient wants, he/she has to make decisions for that patient and may find this role more difficult.
         (c) Because the situations that require decisions based on these documents are often required to be made during hospitalizations, the acute dialysis RN and the patient's nephrologist are most likely to be involved.
      (8) If a patient expresses a wish in writing of "Do Not Resuscitate," staff is restrained from performing CPR or notifying EMS if the patient experiences a cardiopulmonary arrest in the dialysis facility or in any other setting (Hijazi & Holley, 2003).
      (9) For patients with CKD, the principle of autonomy ensures that they have the right to make decisions about initiating treatment and the method of treatment they wish to undergo.
         (a) The professional staff members have the obligation to provide accurate and objective information to the patient so he/she can make an autonomous and informed decision.
         (b) A useful guide in this area is the Renal Physician's Association's Shared Decision Making in the Appropriate Initiation and Withdrawal from Dialysis (RPA, 2010). The recommendation summary and a tool kit are available for free download at this link: http://www.renalmd.org/End-Stage-Renal-Disease/
      (10) For the transplant patient, the principle of autonomy is the underpinning of the living donor's consent and the recipient's willingness to receive the donation. Autonomy is also the ethics principle supporting an adult's expression of willingness to be an organ donor at the time of death and supports the legality of the signed donor card.
5. *Paternalism* (*parentalism*): principle that supports the right of others to make decisions for a competent adult based on belief that the other has

greater knowledge, objectiveness, or abilities, and is acting in the best interest of the individual. This principle allows for conservators or proxies to be legally appointed to act in the best interest of another. In the interest of gender neutrality, the term *parentalism* will be used in this discussion.

a. Historically, parentalism (telling patients what is best for them) was seen by physicians as their obligation and accepted by patients because they had such little knowledge of medicine, disease, and the interventions available to them.
   (1) In the past 50 years, a paradigm shift in patient autonomy, empowerment, and knowledge has occurred, decreasing the acceptance and use of this ethics principle in the United States.
   (2) The practice of parentalism remains dominant in healthcare settings in many other countries/cultures.
b. When applied in Western healthcare settings, physicians or other health professionals may be unaware of their use of parentalism when patient decision making is required.
   (1) Healthcare professionals may demonstrate parentalism because of their cultural influences or due to training received in historical models.
   (2) Outdated nursing "training" may have promoted parentalism.
c. Family and significant others may also exercise parentalism to influence patient wishes or decision making; some patients may struggle against such family or significant other involvement while others expect and welcome it.
d. Application to treatment of CKD stages 1 to 5.
   (1) Parentalism may occur in situations with staff, patients, or families in the treatment setting.
   (2) Staff members need to identify whether they or others are trying to influence or make decisions for the patient and intervene to protect the patient's autonomy if the influence seems unwelcome.
   (3) Staff members also need to determine whether the patient is accepting of parentalistic behaviors.
   (4) Parentalism may lead to the failure to provide sufficient information for each patient with CKD to make his or her own choice of treatment modality.
   (5) Parentalism practiced by both healthcare professionals and the patient's significant others may be one reason for the preponderance of in-center hemodialysis as a KRT (Sullivan, 2010).
   (6) Parentalism (from parents or guardians) is appropriate for pediatric patients facing the initiation of dialysis or transplantation.
      (a) May become a source of contention as the child becomes older and more autonomous (e.g., teenager). Astute staff evaluation and intervention may be required to balance the parentalism and autonomy principles for everyone involved.
      (b) Parentalistic behaviors and decisions by professionals on behalf of pediatric patients and their parents/guardians are problematic and require close observation and interventions to prevent their application to care.
      (c) The most extreme form of parentalism occurs when healthcare professionals legally intervene to prevent family/patient decision making.
         i. Court cases that ask for parents to be relieved of their ability to make healthcare decisions for a child are always complex and contentious.
         ii. Generally represent a failure of communication or of the formal processes used in ethical decision making.
   (7) Parentalism is appropriate and necessary for those patients and families or chosen others to act on behalf of the patient when he/she is unable to make decisions; however, parentalism is often applied informally for minor decisions.
      (a) Staff members should be aware of the need for formal, legal arrangements if decision making on behalf of a patient by others becomes permanent or of major consequence. Staff should also monitor proxy decisions for manipulation or negative impact for the patient.
      (b) In fulfilling the role of patient advocate, staff may need to actively participate in some decision-making situations if the patient has expressed his/her wishes to the staff member.
   (8) Parentalism may also be the underlying principle of some of the "measures of stability" that some transplant programs require patients meet to receive a kidney transplant (e.g., ability to pay for immunosuppressive drugs, assurance of the availability of transportation to and from the transplant center, adequate support system, psychological well-being).

(a) It can be both the patient and the living donor who are treated parentalistically by the transplant team.
(b) With a living donor, the staff may feel and express parentalistic behaviors toward the donor that can be in conflict with the donor's own wishes and decisions. These behaviors can be expressed as rejection of the potential donor as not being a suitable candidate for donation (Spital & Taylor, 2007).

(9) Cultural patterns and the role of family may also play a significant role in the exercise of parentalism within a family group. The healthcare team needs to respect this principle as being an important one to the patient.
(a) Many cultures practice parentalism, allowing the eldest family member to make decisions for younger adults.
(b) For example: a mother decides which of her two adult children on dialysis would receive a compatible kidney from another family member. In addition, the mother tells her son that he may not do peritoneal dialysis (PD) because his sister had experienced multiple problems and complications with PD. The adult son defers to his mother's decision, although he had expressed a desire to undertake PD. This demonstrates the matriarchal culture of this family.

6. *Veracity:* truth-telling; do not lie or withhold the truth.
a. Considered a right in Western culture but may not be universal.
(1) No law guarantees truth-telling in health care.
(2) Because some information about health status, survival, and quality of life cannot be accurately predicted, such information should not be presented as a guarantee or promise to the individual patient.

b. In conjunction with autonomy, veracity is a foundation for the development of required informed consent for the many procedures, surgeries, and treatments that patients undergo.
(1) These legal documents were developed to assure patients are being told the "truth" about what they are to undergo; those truths are identified as risks and benefits (positive and negative outcomes). They must be written in terms patients can understand.
(2) Truth-telling can only be assured if patients have read or have consents read to them. It is a common practice that people sign documents they have not completely read and comprehended. This practice continues to be a problem in health care and elsewhere.
(3) Healthcare professionals should not minimize the process or rush individuals to sign consent forms. It is the professional who is responsible for assuring that patients really understand to what they are consenting.
(4) In transplantation, statements predicting when patients might receive a transplant or potential outcomes of that transplant are embraced by patients as truths or promises. The patients believe they will receive a transplant in the next 6 months because they are told that they are at the "top" of the list.
(5) It is also possible that statements made to patients are misinterpreted because of their need to maintain hope. Their interpretation of what they heard may be different from what was said.

c. Veracity serves as the ethical principle employed in "whistle-blowing."
(1) Defined as telling the truth in the circumstance of illegal activity in the work setting although there is no legal requirement to do so.
(2) This creates a situation of a "should" decision or doing what is right.
(3) For some healthcare workers, doing the right thing outweighs the potential risks. For others, the risks are too great.

d. Lying to patients has been condoned as right/good to prevent harm (nonmaleficence).
(1) Lying about a diagnosis has historically been done to prevent depression or "giving up" by the patient.
(2) While this is now a rare practice in Western health care, it may still occur in other cultures and countries.

e. Application to treatment of CKD stages 1 to 5.
(1) Firm predictions and statements (promises) to patients are difficult to make regarding outcomes, well-being, access to transplantation, best type of therapy, risks of complications, and/or longevity.
(a) Requires staff to remain up-to-date about all available therapies and the most recent data regarding their success and complication rates.
(b) Only reliable data should be shared.
(2) The number of consent/admission documents in dialysis facilities and transplant programs continues to grow.

(a) The task of assuring that patients really understand the content of these documents before signing them is essential.
(b) The staff member obtaining the consents must be qualified to explain the meaning and content of these documents to patients and their significant others.
(3) Whistle-blowing in dialysis and transplantation settings has occurred and generally has been briefly reported only in the popular literature. Studies are not available to document the frequency of such events, the circumstances reported, and the outcomes for the parties involved.

7. *Fidelity*: remaining committed to one's purpose; believing in what one is doing (Bennett, 2004).
   a. Upholding and supporting the philosophy and beliefs of one's employer, the group with whom one is working, and the patients receiving care.
   b. Application to treatment of CKD stages 1 to 5.
      (1) Providing high-quality patient care, maintaining cooperative relationships with colleagues, and assuring that one's performance is reliable and positive in nature.
      (2) The nurse–patient relationship or implied contract for care may be challenged by patient behavior.
      (3) Husted and Husted (2008) provide an example of the patient who states she does not want to continue dialysis but continues to come for treatment because she is frightened by what she has been told about what occurs when dialysis is discontinued. What is the nurse's role and responsibility in this situation?
8. *Utilitarianism*: generally described as the greatest good for the greatest number.
   a. Principle that determines how resources are to be allocated to assure that the largest number of people will benefit from what is available (e.g., finances, access to services or products, and the delivery of those services).
   b. Presumes that all services and products to be allocated are beneficial (Sullivan, 2010; White et al., 2009).
   c. Is usually implemented at a macro (group, community, or population) level rather than at an individual level.
   d. Application to CKD stage 5 treatment: An underlying principle for the passage of PL 92-603 establishing Medicare/Medicaid payment for dialysis and transplantation.
      (1) The choice of which patients would be treated was no longer based on the arbitrary criteria of age, gender, ethnicity, employment, social status, and/or economic status.
      (2) Anyone who might medically benefit from treatment was given access to care; the individual or his/her surrogate could decide whether or not dialysis should be initiated.
      (3) Treatment of CKD stage 5 remains the only federal program funded by Medicare/Medicaid and other insurers that has no socio-economic, demographic, or social restrictions (transplantation of other vital organs funded by Medicare still have some institutional restrictions).
      (4) The underlying ethics principle being applied or challenged is the one regarding allocation of resources when an individual (including a nephrology professional) asks the question, "Why are we dialyzing this person/these people?" (Danis & Hurst, 2009).
9. *Justice as fairness*: distribution of services and products to all based on need.
   a. Requires that some people will receive a greater share based on need than those who do not have as great a need.
   b. May be considered the ethical principle that defines the underpinnings of healthcare insurance (not everyone needs the same quantity of care/payment from the insurance company).
   c. Application to CKD stage 5 treatment: another principle demonstrated by the passage of PL 92-603.
      (1) Equal access to treatment of CKD stage 5 is provided for almost all citizens of the United States via Medicare, Medicaid, and accompanying changes in private health insurance.
      (2) PL 92-603 provides a means to live to those who were dying for lack of money or insurance to pay for treatment.
      (3) May be used to justify the amount of Medicare dollars spent for CKD stage 5 treatment in comparison to other conditions/diseases.

III. History of bioethics in dialysis and transplantation.

A. Use of these treatment technologies preceded the formal definition and organization of the bioethics specialty.
   1. The first successful kidney transplant was done in 1954. In the early years of transplantation, patients

with living related donors sometimes received acute hemodialysis while preparations for transplant surgery were completed.
2. Patients with uremia without living donors sometimes received hemodialysis for short periods, sufficient to get their affairs in order before dying.

B. The first bioethical dilemma in the treatment of kidney disease was identified in 1962 with Dr. Belding Scribner's invention of the external arteriovenous shunt.
   1. This device allowed repeated use of the same blood vessels for hemodialysis.
   2. This in turn allowed for the provision of hemodialysis on a chronic basis, as opposed to the short, temporary time limitations that had been the norm (McCormick, 1993).

C. Once chronic dialysis and kidney transplant were shown to be successful, questions arose regarding how to choose which patients would receive these treatments.
   1. Because resources (e.g., dialysis machines, finances, staff, and facilities) were scarce and had to be allocated, the principles of utilitarianism and/or justice as fairness, beneficence, and nonmaleficence were applied.
   2. Patients were chosen for dialysis based on socioeconomic factors with preference given to:
      a. The middle class.
      b. Working people who paid taxes.
      c. People who were married with children.
      d. Church-going and civic-minded people.
      e. The breadwinner of the family (usually male).
      f. Those who were candidates for kidney transplant (Alexander, 1962).
   3. The University of Washington created a panel of anonymous community representatives to decide which patients would receive treatment.
      a. Their model was replicated at multiple medical centers and hospitals with the resources to provide dialysis.
      b. Home hemodialysis was the only option offered for chronic treatment to provide care to more people (greatest good for the greatest number) (McCormick, 1993).

D. While patient access to dialysis and transplantation was improving, other factors surfaced.
   1. Life-support technologies were successfully employed in trauma situations.
   2. Resuscitation efforts on healthy children and adults were taking place.
   3. These resulted in the need to redefine death.
   4. Brain death was defined and led to a greater number of deceased kidney donors and a concomitant increase in the number of kidney transplants.

E. Through the efforts of nephrologists and other physicians, the National Kidney Foundation, patients and their families, and Congressmen from several states, PL 92-603 became law in 1972. It extended Medicare coverage to patients diagnosed with CKD stage 5 (at the time called ESRD). Based on the ethical principles of utilitarianism and justice as fairness, this law not only resolved some of the ethical dilemmas of patient selection, but also created new ones.

IV. Bioethical dilemmas in the treatment of CKD stage 5.

A. Over the years, the treatment of CKD stage 5 (dialysis and transplantation) has been presented as an example of bioethical dilemmas for patients, healthcare professionals, the healthcare community, and even the general population in various texts, articles, and professional discussions (Gronlund et al., 2011).

B. The public, patients, and nephrology professionals (e.g., physicians, nurses, social workers, psychiatrists, and ethicists) began identifying, discussing, and resolving some of the bioethical dilemmas as early as 1962.
   1. An article in *LIFE* magazine in 1962, "They Decide Who Lives, Who Dies: Medical Miracle and a Moral Burden of a Small Committee," made the medical community and the general public aware of the "ethical" dilemma of patient selection for the limited resource of hemodialysis at one of the first dialysis clinics in the United States (Alexander, 1962).
   2. George Schreiner, an early nephrologist, edited a monograph in 1966 for the CIBA Foundation titled *Ethics in Medical Progress.* One chapter addressed "Problems of Ethics in Relation to Haemo-dialysis and Transplantation" (Wolstenholme & O'Connor, 1966).
   3. Fox and Swazey's (1974) *The Courage to Fail: A Social View of Organ Transplants and Dialysis* documented a number of ethical dilemmas identified via interviews with patients, pioneering nephrologists, and transplant surgeons.
   4. Discussions of ethical dilemmas were a frequent topic at regional meetings held around the country, often cosponsored by ANNA (then known as the American Association of Nephrology Nurses and Technicians or AANNT). These meetings provided a vital forum for discussion of ethics issues by practicing

nephrologists, nurses, social workers, dietitians, and dialysis technicians.

C. Causes of bioethical dilemmas.
   1. A bioethical dilemma occurs when individuals and/or groups disagree about a decision or action that has to occur.
   2. Parties involved have different beliefs and opinions based on their personal experiences, religious or social beliefs, or ethical principles.

D. Resolution requires recognition of the different beliefs and opinions and discussion among the parties involved (i.e., healthcare professionals, patient, family, significant others).
   1. In acute care facilities (i.e., hospitals), an ethics committee is usually available to review referrals of ethical dilemmas made by any staff member, patient, or family/surrogate for resolution.
   2. Ethics committees are generally not available to or located within outpatient dialysis facilities.
   3. Ethical issues are often discussed between individual practitioners (e.g., physician/nurse, physician/social worker, nurse/social worker) and may occur during routinely scheduled patient care conferences or other staff meetings.
      a. In the past, patients and family or surrogates/significant others may not have been included in such discussions, but current regulations expect a more patient-centered approach, which demands that the patient and his/her significant other(s) be included in routine discussions as well as any time an ethical dilemma is identified.
      b. The healthcare providers should not presume to represent the patient's wishes in any care setting, whether inpatient or outpatient.
   4. If an agreement cannot be reached among the involved parties, a third party may need to be consulted. A bioethicist can serve as a consultant/advisor in assisting the parties to resolve the dilemma.
   5. Final resolution may be made in the court system if no agreement can be reached.

E. Guidance for initiation of a formal process for decision making in the dialysis, transplant and/or hospital setting (American Kidney Fund, 2014; Jonsen et al., 2006).
   1. Identify all the interested parties.
      a. Patient, family, and significant others.
      b. Nephrologist.
      c. RNs.
      d. Social worker.
      e. Bioethics expert. Note that hospital settings frequently have an ethics committee that can provide assistance.
   2. If persons are not familiar with the process, an introduction to the principles and ways decisions may be made will be necessary.
   3. Which principle has greatest influence/weight in the decision making? The Western healthcare system generally gives greater weight to the patient's wishes (autonomy) in the resolution of bioethical dilemmas.

F. Use of principles for the resolution of dilemmas.
   1. Beneficence and/or nonmaleficence. Determine whether the benefits of treatment outweigh the harms.
      a. Patients often weigh these two principles as they make decisions about discontinuation of treatment.
         (1) Patients may talk about their "good" days vs. "bad" days. When the number of "bad" days exceeds the number of "good" days, they may consider discontinuation of dialysis.
         (2) Patients who consider "suffering" as a part of life will likely not employ the principles of beneficence/nonmaleficence in their thinking or decision making about treatment and may not be receptive to discussions regarding discontinuation of treatment. They also may not see futility in their condition and would not consider discontinuation of treatment.
   2. Autonomy.
      a. Patients may legally make all decisions about their care if they are competent, of legal age, or an emancipated minor.
         (1) Dialysis staff members must assess patients at the time of admission and throughout their care for evidence of competency (ability to make their own decisions).
         (2) They must also assess whether patients have or need to have a Power of Attorney for Health Care (Lorenz et al., 2008).
      b. If dialysis staff members are concerned about patient competence, they are obligated to pursue referrals for legal protection of the patient.
      c. If there is concern that a patient's autonomy is being limited by family/significant others or health professionals, this should be considered an ethical dilemma; investigation, discussion, and intervention are indicated. In some cases, legal action may be required.
      d. The choice to discontinue treatment may be the maximum expression of autonomy by the patient on dialysis or with a transplant (Fassett et al., 2011; Miller, 1999; Tamura et al., 2010).
      e. In the early days of dialysis, stopping treatment would be socially, emotionally, and legally

interpreted as suicide, affecting the patient's religious life, and causing problems with life insurance payments. Some patients may still hold the belief that discontinuing treatment is a suicidal act; insurance companies have become more enlightened about the principles of autonomy and futility (ANNA, n.d.).

f. Patient autonomy may be expressed by a patient's unwillingness to undergo placement of a permanent vascular access. While staff may see this as a dilemma (perhaps due to externally-imposed performance goals), it is really not an ethical dilemma but represents the patient's expression of autonomy and needs to be respected.

g. Patient behaviors (e.g., nonadherence) may also be considered as an expression of autonomy if the patient has an understanding of his/her behaviors. The behaviors may be thought of as a dilemma (nonethical) with the understanding that the patient has the right to behave as he/she wishes if it causes no direct harm to others (Ripley, 2009).

h. In pediatric dialysis and transplant care, issues of patient and/or family autonomy in decision making may be more challenging (Currier, 1994).
   (1) Because of laws related to prevention of child abuse and protection of minors, decisions about the treatment of children are more likely to become a legal matter if a conflict occurs. These conflicts could be between family members, parent and child, or family and healthcare providers.
   (2) Discontinuation of treatment is especially problematic. While the legal age of consent in the United States is 18, many pediatric professionals advocate that children may have enough understanding of their illness and treatment to express their wishes in a situation of a dilemma and decision making and will weigh their wishes in the process. Conflicts between parents (and other significant family members) are also likely to occur and be expressed in legal ways (e.g., custody fights or legal surrogacy requests) (Doyal & Henning, 1994; Lantos & Warody, 2012).

i. In kidney transplantation, autonomy is the pivotal ethical principle underlying the availability of both living and deceased donor organs (Simmons, 1977). It is the principle employed to support the legal right of organ donation per:
   (1) The wishes of the potential donor via a signed card/document.
   (2) Confirmation of the wishes of the potential donor by legal next of kin.
   (3) Decision making by the next of kin on behalf of the potential donor.

j. The principle of autonomy also is paramount to a living donor giving consent for removal of a kidney for transplant to another individual. The concern of staff regarding whether these are autonomous or coerced decisions continues to be an ethical issue/dilemma for transplant staff and patients (Joffe, 2007; Mazaris et al., 2009).

3. The principle of futility, as determined by the patient, may also be employed to allow the patient to forgo or discontinue treatment without any legal repercussions. Patients who do not weigh the beneficence/nonmaleficence of the outcomes of treatment or who believe that suffering is part of living may not embrace the principle of futility as the healthcare team members might.

4. Parentalism: the most powerful person decides. This is often seen by patient or family as the physician, but it can also be the most vocal person, the closest next of kin, or the eldest family member.
   a. Has become a less acceptable method in Western/U.S. culture.
   b. Denies patients their autonomy.
   c. If the patient is an elder, the possibility of elder abuse may arise when other adults are caring for and making decisions for the elder person.
      (1) Major ethical decisions in these circumstances should be carefully analyzed to protect the patient from abuse (physical, social, financial), harm, or untimely death.
      (2) Elder abuse is a reportable offense in many states.
   d. Historically, parentalism has also been used in violation of the principle of veracity.
      (1) Family members and physicians may choose not to provide patients with information about a "bad" diagnosis.
      (2) The physician and family would collaborate in determining what, how, and if treatment would be given.
   e. Patients may give consent and/or arrange for parentalism.
      (1) Competent patients can tell the physician/healthcare team to "do what they think is best."
      (2) Without a discussion of their wishes with a surrogate, patients may sign a Durable Power of Attorney for Health Care or POLST assigning the surrogate to make healthcare decisions on their behalf.

f. For patients (pediatric or adult) on dialysis or with transplants who may suffer from altered mental status and/or an acute condition that prevents active participation in decision making, parentalism may be appropriate. For example:
   (1) Decisions regarding initiation or discontinuance of dialysis that may be made by family.
   (2) Decisions regarding treatment of other medical conditions or illnesses (e.g., cardiac surgery, treatment of cancer, and treatment of sepsis or cardiac arrest situations) may be made by family.

g. Parentalism is often employed when physicians make strong recommendations about a specific treatment modality or do not provide adequate information or opportunity for patients to make informed, autonomous choices.

h. Nurses, especially those working in acute dialysis and who have spent time with the patient and family, may/should serve as the patient's advocate in acute care situations. It may be appropriate to recommend consultation from the ethics committee when conflict arises or there is evidence that patient's wishes could be violated.

i. A continuing legal concern is that family members/surrogates may make decisions to benefit themselves (e.g., inheritance, income, burden of care) that are not in best interest of the patient.

5. Veracity and fidelity: these principles apply to all healthcare providers including ancillary staff and to patients, their families, and significant others.
   a. For the healthcare facility, fidelity includes maintaining its commitment to the delivery of high-quality care in a timely fashion.
   b. The "Patient Rights and Responsibilities" documents that patients are provided and asked to sign in various healthcare settings address some aspects of both the patients' and the facility's promises related to veracity and fidelity.
   c. Many of the actions requested of patients are determined by an agreement of veracity (e.g., providing information) and fidelity (e.g., maintaining a dialysis schedule, following the plan of care, taking the ordered immunosuppressive medications, and keeping follow-up appointments).
   d. Veracity and fidelity are also codified in informed consent documents that patients are asked to sign. It is the staff's obligation to ensure that patients understand the information.
   e. May be applied to staff giving information about treatment modalities. The information and presentation must be clear, accurate, and without bias.

6. Utilitarianism and justice as fairness are ethics principles applied to delivery of care for CKD stage 5.
   a. Generally beyond the level of individual facilities, staff, and patients.
   b. Employed by various agencies including insurance companies, state and federal governments, and other interested parties (e.g., advocacy groups or foundations, patient groups, professional groups).
   c. One continuing dilemma defined by these principles is regarding the provision of care to undocumented (and frequently unfunded) immigrants.
      (1) Facilities throughout the United States have been confronted by this dilemma and have arrived at resolutions in various ways generally dependent on state laws and regulations about health care.
      (2) This results in a problem of inequity because treatment is dependent on the state in which the patient resides (Campbell et al., 2010).

7. Interested individuals can be activists and supporters of movements and changes needed to assure justice for patients. ANNA plays a significant role in lobbying and supporting efforts to assure justice as fairness for patients with kidney disease.

V. Summary.

A. The nephrology community has been a leader in the identification and resolution of ethical dilemmas.

B. Nephrology nurses need to remain informed and active at the patient care level, the administrative level of the hospital and dialysis facility, and at political and governmental levels to identify the ethical principles underlying or potentially being violated by actions being proposed or adopted relevant to nursing and nephrology care.

C. Nephrology nurses also need to be aware of new technologies and treatments being developed that can create new ethical problems or dilemmas for both the nephrology patient population and healthcare professionals.

D. Ethical issues and dilemmas being faced today and into the future include:
   1. Treatment reimbursement (allocation of resources).

2. The continued growth of the CKD stage 5 population, including the indigent and noncitizens/residents who cannot pay for their medications/treatments (justice as fairness).
3. Fair reimbursement for new methods of delivery of dialysis, such as home hemodialysis (allocation of resources).
4. An increased number of patients desiring transplantation in the face of a scarcity of donor organs and changes in kidney donor sources (e.g., potential payment for kidney donation [allocation of resources, justice as fairness]).

E. While these are major ethical issues, individual ethical dilemmas may still occur in any nephrology setting. Nephrology nurses must be aware of and sensitive to any potential ethical dilemmas that the patients may be facing.

SECTION C
Leadership and Management

Glenda M. Payne • Nancy B. Pierce • Lillian A. Pryor

I. All nurses are leaders. One of the findings of the IOM Future of Nursing (FON) report (2010) was that nurses need to take leadership roles in all settings to meet the demands of our changing healthcare system.

A. A key finding of the FON report is the need to recognize the importance of lifelong learning. Padmasree Warrior, the chief technology officer of Cisco, is quoted by the *Huffington Post* in 2011 as believing that "the ability to learn is the most important quality a leader can have" (Bosker, 2011).

B. Sheryl Sandberg's *Lean In* (2013), subtitled *Women, Work and the Will to Lead*, describes the importance of women recognizing their value and "leaning in" to responsibility rather than sitting back. This axiom can be applied by every nurse (male as well as female) as it becomes evermore important to bring nursing's voice to the table as healthcare issues are addressed.

C. Sandberg reports (2013) personal communication from the dean and associate dean of Harvard Business School: "Leadership is about making others better as a result of your presence and making sure that impact lasts in your absence" (p. 157). With nursing's traditional values of helping others, this view of leadership is a natural fit.

D. ANNA and ANA offer many online resources to develop personal leadership skills. The following sections provide a starting point.

II. Management responsibilities.

A. Staff satisfaction: One of the most important responsibilities of a leader is to assure staff satisfaction. The goal is to create excited and engaged employees who look forward to coming to work, do a great job, and treat patients well. Tye (2014) discusses the value of invisible architecture: "Invisible architecture is to the soul of your organization what physical architecture is to its body. Invisible architecture, not the buildings, determines whether you are a good healthcare facility, a great healthcare facility or just another healthcare facility" (p 14). This invisible architecture must include valuing and developing the following staff characteristics: commitment, engagement, passion, initiative, stewardship, belonging, fellowship, and pride.
1. Importance to an organization.
    a. Staff satisfaction creates good patient satisfaction. Employees' needs must be met before they can focus on meeting and exceeding patient needs.
    b. Engaged and satisfied employees are more productive, better stewards of limited resources, use fewer sick-leave days, do a better job, and are more creative and resourceful. Engaged and satisfied employees are self-empowered to problem-solve. They are "fully present physically as well as emotionally" (Tye, 2014, p. 19).
        (1) "Always treat your employees exactly like you want them to treat your best customers. You can buy a person's hand, but you can't buy his heart. You can buy his back, but you can't buy his brain. That's where the creativity is, his ingenuity, his resourcefulness" (Covey, 2005a, p. 58).
        (2) "You can hold people accountable for showing up on time and for fulfilling the terms of their job descriptions, but you cannot hold them accountable for being committed and engaged. You cannot hold people accountable for caring. It takes a spirit of ownership for those things to happen" (Tye, 2014, p. 16). Development of this spirit of ownership in employees is the key to the organization's success.
    c. Lower turnover costs.
        (1) According to Boushey & Glynn (2012), the cost of turnover can be as much as 20% of an employee's annual salary. Their review of 30 case studies in 11 of the most relevant

research papers published between 1992 and 2007 on the cost of turnover demonstrated the cost to business is about one-fifth of an employee's annual salary to replace that worker.

(a) Direct costs include searching, recruiting, and training.

(b) Indirect costs can include reduced quality of care while covering the loss, decreased or disrupted continuity of care, reduced morale of those left behind, less productivity for a period of time during and after training, increased workload of others, and loss of historical knowledge.

2. What is important to employees (Studer, 2003).
   a. Purpose. Employees want to believe their organization has the right purpose and to feel proud of their organization and leaders. Managers who make themselves look good at the expense of senior leadership do a disservice to the employees as senior leaders represent "purpose" to employees.
      (1) Leaders must avoid a "we/they" culture, and proudly and enthusiastically support senior management. If employees feel good about senior leaders, they feel good about the organization.
      (2) Employees' commitment to values, vision, and mission is an important step in ensuring a spirit of ownership (Tye, 2014).
   b. Worthwhile work. The employees must value their work, as must their leader. It is the responsibility of the leader to periodically acknowledge this value to the employees. This increases engagement, and engaged employees have passion – loving their work and letting it show (Tye, 2014).
   c. Making a difference: People want to make a difference in life. Getting rewarding results fuels their passion and motivates them to continue to persevere and seek more results. As they make a difference in patients' lives, the patients' satisfaction rises.
      (1) Engaged employees take initiative to see what needs to be done and take action to get it done. They are self-empowered. "Some of the most influential leaders in an organization don't have a management title. They are leaders because they see what needs to be done, they're willing to take the initiative, and they're able to influence others to work with them" (Tye 2014, p. 126.).
      (2) Tye (2014) also states: "Leaders must often follow those whom one is supposed to be leading. Indeed, when there is a culture of ownership, leaders are often followers and followers are often leaders" (p. 15).
3. Strategies should "focus on the positive." Leaders need to train themselves to focus on what is "right" rather than "wrong" and share those "wins" throughout the organization. To collect the stories about those "wins," leaders need to routinely round with employees.
   a. According to Studer (2003), "Rounding for Outcomes" is the number one action to drive improved staff satisfaction (see Figures 1.1 and 1.2).
      (1) Through rounding, employees develop a good relationship with their supervisor.
         (a) According to Studer (2003), "a poor relationship with the supervisor is the reason 39% of staff leave their jobs!" (p. 143).
         (b) Gardner and Walton (2011) report that the results of their study on nephrology nurse retention and job satisfaction found that nurses were frustrated when not recognized as valued team members.
         (c) Rounding with staff nurses provides an opportunity to recognize good work.
      (2) Studer (2003) lists the following qualities that staff members look for in a supervisor.
         (a) A good relationship.
         (b) Approachability.
         (c) Willingness to work side by side.
         (d) Efficient systems.
         (e) Training and development.
         (f) Tools and equipment to do the job.
         (g) Appreciation.
      (3) Studer (2003) suggests five basic questions to use when rounding with staff (p. 144).

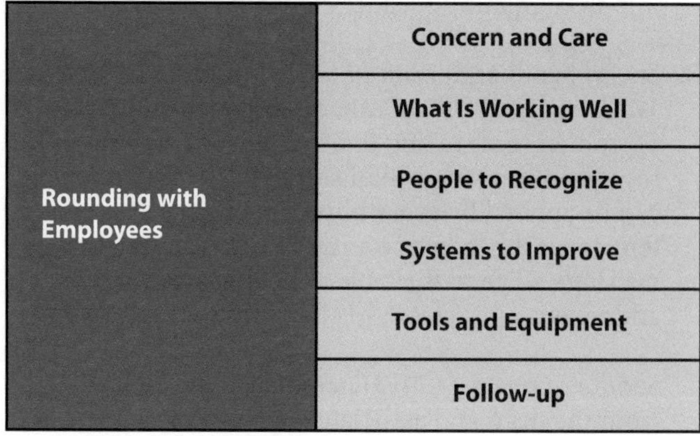

Figure 1.1. Communication flow for rounding on employees. When you are rounding, your talking points should follow a specific flow. This keeps you on track, helps you manage the encounter, and encourages you to keep conversations consistent from employee to employee. Adapted from *The Nurse Leader Handbook*. Copyright 2010, the Studer Group. All rights reserved. Used with permission.

StuderGroup®

ROUNDING for Outcomes STAFF UNIT ______________ Manager ______________

Staff Member/Date	Relationship Learning	What is working well today?	Staff recognized and why	Departments recognized and why	Physicians recognized and why	Systems needing improvements & ideas to fix	Tools and equipment needed
1.							
2.							
3.							
4.							
5.							
6.							

Figure 1.2. Sample Rounding Tool designed by the Studer Group (2010, p. 27). *Used with permission from the Studer Group.*

(a) Tell me what is working well today.
(b) Are there any individuals whom I should be recognizing?
(c) Are there any physicians whom I should be recognizing? (If appropriate.)
(d) Is there anything we can do better?
(e) Do you have the tools and equipment to do your work?

b. Act on and follow through with the information received during rounding. This demonstrates that employees' input makes a difference and increases their job satisfaction.

(1) Provide positive feedback regarding the positive stories ("wins") that were collected.

(a) Let each person mentioned (e.g., coworkers, physicians, out-of-department workers, etc.) know his/her action was appreciated and commented on by a specific staff member during rounding.
(b) This positive feedback rewards and recognizes others, and the recognized behavior will get repeated. Studer (2003) calls this "Success Builds Success" (p. 145). People subsequently feel that their work is worthwhile because others appreciated it, and they will repeat that good work.
(c) "Leadership is communicating to people their worth and potential so clearly that they come to see it in themselves" (Covey, 2005b, p. 98).

(2) Obtain any tools and equipment identified as needed so people can do their jobs efficiently.
(3) Work to correct identified systems issues.
(4) Communicate results from rounding. See Department "Stop Light Report" example (Figure 1.3).

(a) What has been fixed?
(b) What is in process and expected completion date?
(c) What are you unable to do, along with the reason why?

SPOTLIGHT REPORT

Note: The spotlight report is a way to communicate in writing how the ideas/concerns harvested in rounding are dealt with. It is excellent to post on communication boards. Green Light items are things that have been addressed and are complete. Yellow Light items are things in progress. Red Light items are those issues or ideas that cannot be done with the reason why.

To think about as you construct your report:

- Format the report in a way that is meaningful to you and your direct reports.
- This report is a reflection of you and should be neat and orderly.
- These are an important way to communicate with your direct reports. Make sure each item is understandable to someone who might read it "cold."
- Keep your fonts the same style and size.
- Provide enough information that allows the reader understanding.

Department/Unit/Clinic:	Date:

GREEN/COMPLETE	YELLOW/WORK IN PROGRESS	RED/CAN'T COMPLETE AT THIS TIME AND HERE'S WHY

StuderGroup © 2014 Malcolm Baldrige National Quality Award 2010 Award Recipient

Figure 1.3. Sample of a Stop Light Report from the Studer Group. Adapted from *The Nurse Leader Handbook*. Copyright 2010, the Studer Group. All rights reserved. Used with permission.

c. The power of sending out thank-you notes (Studer, 2003).
   (1) It is very powerful to send a personal thank-you note to an employee's home. This method also informs the family of your appreciation.
   (2) Having a senior management leader co-sign and comment on the thank-you note makes even more of an impact.
   (3) Making thank-you note writing a routine part of weekly management responsibilities is important to success.
      (a) Make sure each employee gets a note periodically; everyone needs to know that their work is important and noticed.
      (b) Make a chart to keep track of notes written or need to be written, when, and the reason.
      (c) Set aside a period of time every week to write these notes.
      (d) The note does not need to be long but should be specific to the situation, including who commented and what was achieved or appreciated.

B. Effective communication with staff. It is important that organizations have transparency and employees are kept continually updated about current information. A variety of processes can be used.
   1. One effective way to present communication to staff is group messaging using the five "Pillars for

The 5 Pillars of Healthcare Success				
Service	**Quality**	**People**	**Finance**	**Growth**
• Delighted patients • Reduced legal expenses • Reduced malpractice expense	• Improved clinical outcomes – decreased nosocomial infections • Reduced lengths of stay • Reduced re-admits • Reduced medication errors	• Reduced turnover • Reduced vacancies • Reduced agency costs • Reduced PRN • Reduced overtime • Delighted A-Team members	• Increased bed turns • Reduced vacancies • Reduced agency costs • Reduced PRN • Reduced overtime • Reduced physicals and cost to orient	• Higher volume • Increased revenue • Decreased left without treatment in the ED • Reduced outpatient no-shows • Increased physician activity

Figure 1.4. Pillar management: Populating the pillars with defined goals. Adapted from *The Nurse Leader Handbook*. Copyright 2010, the Studer Group. All rights reserved. Used with permission.

Healthcare Success." The pillars represent facility goals (Studer Group, 2010). A bulletin board with postings under each pillar will demonstrate to the employees how the facility is meeting important organizational goals. Examples of pillars and typical postings under each are noted below (see Figures 1.4 and 1.5).

a. Pillar #1: Service. The goal is delighted patients. Postings might include:
   (1) Most recent patient satisfaction surveys.
   (2) Aggregate In-center Hemodialysis Consumer Assessment of Healthcare Providers and Systems (ICH CAHPS) scores.
   (3) Examples of thank-you notes from patients and families.
   (4) Specific service standards the organization is focusing on for improvement.

b. Pillar #2: Quality. The goal is improved clinical outcomes. Postings might include:
   (1) Progress on specific process improvement projects related to quality and safety.
   (2) Patient clinical outcomes for anemia, bone disease, vascular access, etc.
   (3) Outcome measures and scores related to CMS' ESRD financial incentives, e.g., the Quality Incentive Program (QIP).

c. Pillar #3: People. The goal is employee satisfaction. Postings might include:
   (1) Upcoming employee educational events.
      (a) Mandatory competency education schedules.

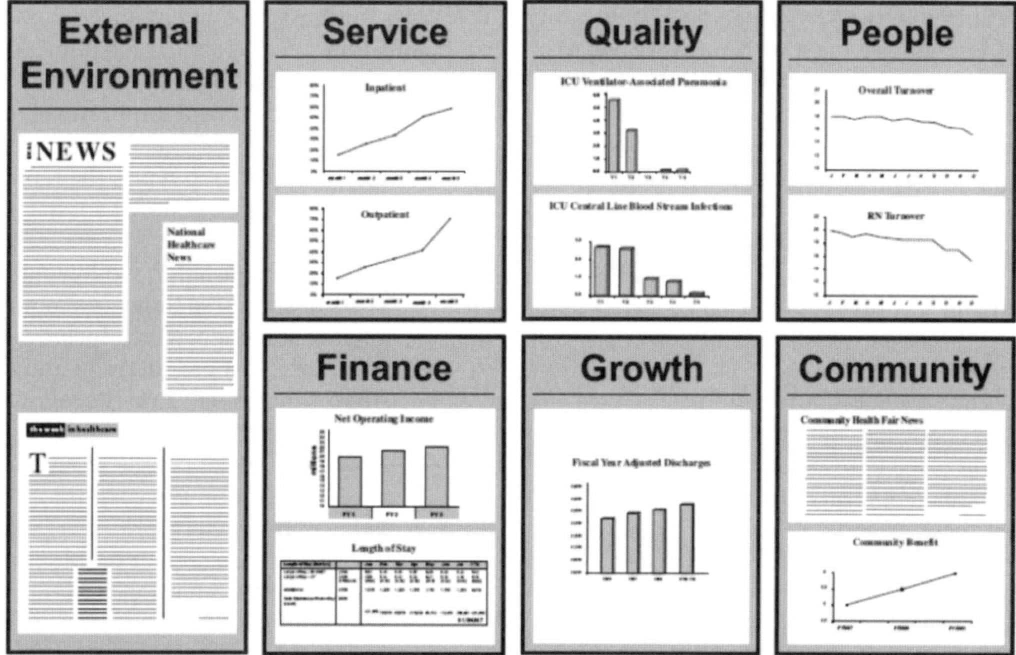

Figure 1.5. Communication Board Example. Adapted from *The Nurse Leader Handbook*. Copyright 2010, the Studer Group. All rights reserved. Used with permission.

(b) Upcoming continuing education opportunities and how much organizational financial support is available.
(2) Benefits information.
(3) Staff satisfaction survey results.
(4) Stories that celebrate specific staff members' awards and recognition.
(5) Information about new physicians and new employees.
(6) Employee turnover rate.

d. Pillar # 4: Finance. The goal is financial success. Postings might include:
(1) Data concerning the current financial state of the organization or department.
(2) Departmental or budgetary concerns (productivity numbers, etc.).

e. Pillar #5: Growth. The goal is to increase or augment needed services. Postings might include:
(1) Data regarding growth goals such as:
(a) Percentage of the patient population that is on home hemodialysis and/or peritoneal dialysis versus in-center hemodialysis.
(b) The number of transplants accomplished in the last quarter.
(2) Number of patients attending CKD education sessions.

2. Departmental newsletters can be printed or sent electronically to employees (see Figure 1.6).
a. Celebrate successes and awards.
b. Announce upcoming events and staff birthdays.
c. Recognize organizational people who have been featured in the newspaper, on TV, etc.

3. Daily huddles with staff at a set time every day for communication and team building. These huddles should not last more than 10 to 15 minutes; a theme can be chosen for certain days of the week. Suggested topics for huddles include:
a. Begin each meeting with a safety story.
b. What is going well; include celebrations.
c. Share stories to reinforce organizational values and provide examples of high performance and exceeding customer/patient/family expectations.
d. Devote time for staff appreciation.
e. Potential challenges for the day and a quick update on plans to resolve them.
f. Quick status report on current quality improvement projects.
g. Rumors that need to be addressed.
h. "Wildcard day." Discuss an issue that may be a source of frustration for the staff. This may result in the need to schedule another meeting if there is a need for more discussion or to form a resolution team.

4. Effective staff meetings.
a. Prepare a written agenda ahead of time to include outcome objectives for the meeting.
(1) Include any data that will be reviewed and discussed at the meeting such as quality outcome measures and goals with historical data.
(2) Provide a copy of the agenda to all attendees.
b. Schedule at a routine day and time of month, (e.g., second Tuesday at 10 a.m.) so staff can plan ahead to attend.
c. Include all members of the interdisciplinary team: physicians, social workers, dietitians, nurses, technicians, biomedical staff, pharmacists, etc.
d. Include time to celebrate successes and share positive stories.
e. Start on time and end on time, or early if the meeting objectives have been met.

5. Employee forums.
a. Quarterly updates from senior level management regarding organizational goals and objectives as well as celebration of achievements.
b. Provides an opportunity for staff and senior leaders to get to know one another.
(1) Provide sufficient time for a question and answer session.
(2) Consider providing a written handout for staff.
(3) Make it fun. Provide food and door prizes!

C. Selecting and retaining talented employees. The leader must assure that employees hired have the talents they need to get the job done and are a right fit for the organizational culture.
1. Financial and clinical implications for hiring the right person.
a. For healthcare job types, the replacement costs can be as high as 20% of annual pay (Cleaver, 2013).
b. Blackwell reported the following in 2011: "...It costs nearly three times an employee's salary to replace someone, which includes recruitment, severance, lost productivity, and lost opportunities" (p. 23). The following turnover rates are cited by Blackwell (2011, p. 23):
(1) Over 50% of people recruited into an organization leave within 2 years.
(2) Approximately 50% of organizations experience regular problems with employee retention.
(3) Nearly 70% of organizations report that staff turnover has negative financial impact due to the costs of recruiting, hiring, training a replacement employee, and the

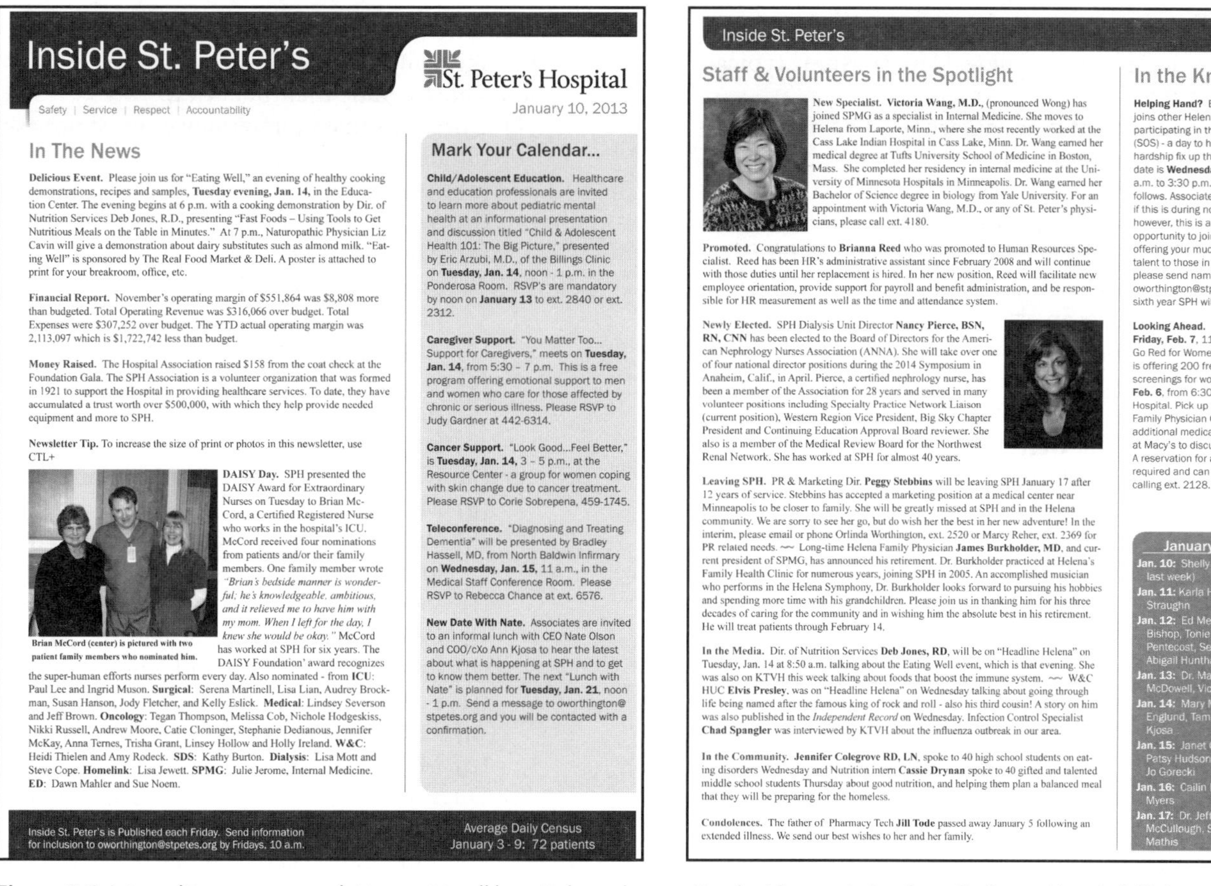

Inside St. Peter's

Safety | Service | Respect | Accountability

St. Peter's Hospital

January 10, 2013

In The News

Delicious Event. Please join us for "Eating Well," an evening of healthy cooking demonstrations, recipes and samples, **Tuesday evening, Jan. 14,** in the Education Center. The evening begins at 6 p.m. with a cooking demonstration by Dir. of Nutrition Services Deb Jones, R.D., presenting "Fast Foods – Using Tools to Get Nutritious Meals on the Table in Minutes." At 7 p.m., Naturopathic Physician Liz Cavin will give a demonstration about dairy substitutes such as almond milk. "Eating Well" is sponsored by The Real Food Market & Deli. A poster is attached to print for your breakroom, office, etc.

Financial Report. November's operating margin of $551,864 was $8,808 more than budgeted. Total Operating Revenue was $316,066 over budget. Total Expenses were $307,252 over budget. The YTD actual operating margin was 2,113,097 which is $1,722,742 less than budget.

Money Raised. The Hospital Association raised $158 from the coat check at the Foundation Gala. The SPH Association is a volunteer organization that was formed in 1921 to support the Hospital in providing healthcare services. To date, they have accumulated a trust worth over $500,000, with which they help provide needed equipment and more to SPH.

Newsletter Tip. To increase the size of print or photos in this newsletter, use CTL+

DAISY Day. SPH presented the DAISY Award for Extraordinary Nurses on Tuesday to Brian McCord, a Certified Registered Nurse who works in the hospital's ICU. McCord received four nominations from patients and/or their family members. One family member wrote *"Brian's bedside manner is wonderful; he's knowledgeable, ambitious, and it relieved me to have him with my mom. When I left for the day, I knew she would be okay."* McCord has worked at SPH for six years. The DAISY Foundation' award recognizes the super-human efforts nurses perform every day. Also nominated - from **ICU**: Paul Lee and Ingrid Muson. **Surgical**: Serena Martinell, Lisa Lian, Audrey Brockman, Susan Hanson, Jody Fletcher, and Kelly Eslick. **Medical**: Lindsey Severson and Jeff Brown. **Oncology**: Tegan Thompson, Melissa Cob, Nichole Hodgeskiss, Nikki Russell, Andrew Moore, Catie Cloninger, Stephanie Dedianous, Jennifer McKay, Anna Ternes, Trisha Grant, Linsey Hollow and Holly Ireland. **W&C**: Heidi Thielen and Amy Rodeck. **SDS**: Kathy Burton. **Dialysis**: Lisa Mott and Steve Cope. **Homelink**: Lisa Jewett. **SPMG**: Julie Jerome, Internal Medicine. **ED**: Dawn Mahler and Sue Noem.

Brian McCord (center) is pictured with two patient family members who nominated him.

Mark Your Calendar...

Child/Adolescent Education. Healthcare and education professionals are invited to learn more about pediatric mental health at an informational presentation and discussion titled "Child & Adolescent Health 101: The Big Picture," presented by Eric Arzubi, M.D., of the Billings Clinic on **Tuesday, Jan. 14**, noon - 1 p.m. in the Ponderosa Room. RSVP's are mandatory by noon on **January 13** to ext. 2840 or ext. 2312.

Caregiver Support. "You Matter Too... Support for Caregivers," meets on **Tuesday, Jan. 14**, from 5:30 – 7 p.m. This is a free program offering emotional support to men and women who care for those affected by chronic or serious illness. Please RSVP to Judy Gardner at 442-6314.

Cancer Support. "Look Good...Feel Better," is **Tuesday, Jan. 14,** 3 – 5 p.m., at the Resource Center - a group for women coping with skin change due to cancer treatment. Please RSVP to Corie Sobrepena, 459-1745.

Teleconference. "Diagnosing and Treating Dementia" will be presented by Bradley Hassell, MD, from North Baldwin Infirmary on **Wednesday, Jan. 15,** 11 a.m., in the Medical Staff Conference Room. Please RSVP to Rebecca Chance at ext. 6576.

New Date With Nate. Associates are invited to an informal lunch with CEO Nate Olson and COO/cXo Ann Kjosa to hear the latest about what is happening at SPH and to get to know them better. The next "Lunch with Nate" is planned for **Tuesday, Jan. 21**, noon - 1 p.m. Send a message to oworthington@stpetes.org and you will be contacted with a confirmation.

Inside St. Peter's is Published each Friday. Send information for inclusion to oworthington@stpetes.org by Fridays, 10 a.m.

Average Daily Census
January 3 - 9: 72 patients

Inside St. Peter's — page 2

Staff & Volunteers in the Spotlight

New Specialist. Victoria Wang, M.D., (pronounced Wong) has joined SPMG as a specialist in Internal Medicine. She moves to Helena from Laporte, Minn., where she most recently worked at the Cass Lake Indian Hospital in Cass Lake, Minn. Dr. Wang earned her medical degree at Tufts University School of Medicine in Boston, Mass. She completed her residency in internal medicine at the University of Minnesota Hospitals in Minneapolis. Dr. Wang earned her Bachelor of Science degree in biology from Yale University. For an appointment with Victoria Wang, M.D., or any of St. Peter's physicians, please call ext. 4180.

Promoted. Congratulations to **Brianna Reed** who was promoted to Human Resources Specialist. Reed has been HR's administrative assistant since February 2008 and will continue with those duties until her replacement is hired. In her new position, Reed will facilitate new employee orientation, provide support for payroll and benefit administration, and be responsible for HR measurement as well as the time and attendance system.

Newly Elected. SPH Dialysis Unit Director **Nancy Pierce, BSN, RN, CNN** has been elected to the Board of Directors for the American Nephrology Nurses Association (ANNA). She will take over one of four national director positions during the 2014 Symposium in Anaheim, Calif., in April. Pierce, a certified nephrology nurse, has been a member of the Association for 28 years and served in many volunteer positions including Specialty Practice Network Liaison (current position), Western Region Vice President, Big Sky Chapter President and Continuing Education Approval Board reviewer. She also is a member of the Medical Review Board for the Northwest Renal Network. She has worked at SPH for almost 40 years.

Leaving SPH. PR & Marketing Dir. **Peggy Stebbins** will be leaving SPH January 17 after 12 years of service. Stebbins has accepted a marketing position at a medical center near Minneapolis to be closer to family. She will be greatly missed at SPH and in the Helena community. We are sorry to see her go, but do wish her the best in her new adventure! In the interim, please email or phone Orlinda Worthington, ext. 2520 or Marcy Reher, ext. 2369 for PR related needs. ~~ Long-time Helena Family Physician **James Burkholder, MD**, and current president of SPMG, has announced his retirement. Dr. Burkholder practiced at Helena's Family Health Clinic for numerous years, joining SPH in 2005. An accomplished musician who performs in the Helena Symphony, Dr. Burkholder looks forward to pursuing his hobbies and spending more time with his grandchildren. Please join us in thanking him for his three decades of caring for the community and in wishing him the absolute best in his retirement. He will treat patients through February 14.

In the Media. Dir. of Nutrition Services **Deb Jones, RD**, will be on "Headline Helena" on Tuesday, Jan. 14 at 8:50 a.m. talking about the Eating Well event, which is that evening. She was also on KTVH this week talking about foods that boost the immune system. ~~ W&C HUC **Elvis Presley**, was on "Headline Helena" on Wednesday talking about going through life being named after the famous king of rock and roll - also his third cousin! A story on him was also published in the *Independent Record* on Wednesday. Infection Control Specialist **Chad Spangler** was interviewed by KTVH about the influenza outbreak in our area.

In the Community. **Jennifer Colegrove RD, LN**, spoke to 40 high school students on eating disorders Wednesday and Nutrition intern **Cassie Drynan** spoke to 40 gifted and talented middle school students Thursday about good nutrition, and helping them plan a balanced meal that they will be preparing for the homeless.

Condolences. The father of Pharmacy Tech **Jill Tode** passed away January 5 following an extended illness. We send our best wishes to her and her family.

In the Know

Helping Hand? Each year SPH joins other Helena organizations in participating in the Spirit of Service (SOS) - a day to help those experiencing hardship fix up their homes. This year's date is **Wednesday, May 28**, from 8:30 a.m. to 3:30 p.m. A picnic for volunteers follows. Associates must use PL time if this is during normal work hours; however, this is a great once-a-year opportunity to join your co-workers offering your much needed time and talent to those in need. To volunteer, please send name and T-shirt size to oworthington@stpetes.org This is the sixth year SPH will be a SOS partner.

Looking Ahead. Mark your calendar for **Friday, Feb. 7**, 11 a.m. - 1:30 p.m for Go Red for Women at Macy's. Wellness is offering 200 free heart health screenings for women on **Thursday, Feb. 6**, from 6:30 - 10:30 a.m. at the Hospital. Pick up results at Go Red. Family Physician Cathy Lay, M.D., and additional medical staff will be available at Macy's to discuss screening results. A reservation for a free screening is required and can be made online or by calling ext. 2128.

January Birthdays

Jan. 10: Shelly Edwards (omitted last week)
Jan. 11: Karla Hardy, Eileen Straughn
Jan. 12: Ed Meardon, Russell Bishop, Tonie Solee, Anna Pentecost, Serena Martinell, Abigail Hunthausen
Jan. 13: Dr. Mark Kreisberg, Janell McDowell, Victoria Kocher
Jan. 14: Mary Mistek, Alvera Englund, Tammy Beattie, Ann Kjosa
Jan. 15: Janet Gill, Paula Mansfield, Patsy Hudson, Kelly Hunt, Marla Jo Gorecki
Jan. 16: Cailin Martello, Heather Myers
Jan. 17: Dr. Jeff Georgia, Cindy McCullough, Sandy Herzog, Lori Mathis

Figure 1.6. Internal two-page newsletter sent to all hospital employees. Used with permission from St. Peters Hospital, Helena, MT.

overtime work of current employees required until the organization can fill the vacant position.

(4) Nearly 70% of organizations report having difficulties in replacing staff.

(5) One new hire in four will leave an organization within 6 months.

c. Don't just hire a body – hire a good fit. If the person is not a good fit, they can negatively impact other employees or leave, wasting the time and resources invested in his/her orientation.

d. Hire for talents needed for the job, positive attitude, and enthusiasm – not just previous clinical experience. Clinical skills can be taught, but it is not possible to change a person's basic personality to fit the job.

2. Interviewing skills.

a. Selection. First prescreen for qualifications for the particular job.

(1) Minimum educational and experience requirements must be met.

(2) Screen for ability to do essential functions and relevance of past schooling and employment to the current opening.

(3) Screen out candidates who have a long history of moving quickly from job to job for no obvious reason.

b. Use a behavioral-type interview (Studer Group, n.d.). The best predictor of how a new employee will function in this position is how they functioned in past jobs.

(1) Can candidates illustrate what they have done previously by describing an event or situation in response to interview questions? What action did the candidates take? What was the result or outcome of the experience?

(2) Listen closely to what the candidates say and look for nonverbal clues about how they actually feel about a question or subject.

(3) Evaluate for manner, motivation, self-expression, responsiveness, integrity, honesty, trustworthiness, temperament, adaptability, interpersonal relations, social skills, growth and development, reaction to authority, maturity, character, judgment, talents, energy, time management, productivity, teamwork, and positive attitude.

(4) It is important to plan your questions and

interview session. Develop a form or template as a guide. Here are some typical questions.
   (a) What types of tasks or jobs have you enjoyed doing in the past and why?
   (b) What did you do in your last job to contribute toward a teamwork environment? Describe how you felt your contributions affected the team.
   (c) Give an example of someone or something that irritated or frustrated you in your past job and how you dealt with this. What was the outcome?
   (d) Who were the best and worst supervisors you have had and why for each?
   (e) What was the toughest problem you faced in your last job and how did you deal with it?
   (f) Describe a situation in which you felt it might be justifiable to break company policy or alter a standard procedure. What did you do?
   (g) Think of a day when you were extremely busy. Describe how you scheduled your time.
   (h) Give me an example of an important goal that had been set for you and describe your success in reaching it.
   (i) Why did you leave your last three jobs?
   (j) When is the last time you were criticized at work? How did you deal with it?
   (k) Describe your personality and your primary motivators.
   (l) If I call your references, what will they tell me about you?
   (m) What kind of environment do you like to work in?
   (n) What are you most proud of?
   (o) When taking on a new task, do you like to have a great deal of feedback and directions at the start, or do you like to try your own approach?
   (p) What are your short and long-term career goals?
   (q) Why should we hire you?
   (r) Do you have questions for me?

c. After the supervisor deems one or more candidates as acceptable for hire, schedule future coworkers to conduct a "peer interview." The coworkers can then make a recommendation for hiring, allowing them to have a voice in the decision. Choose employees who are well-respected leaders and high performers to do the peer interviews. Ensure the peer interviewers are trained regarding legal restrictions on questions that can and cannot be asked, and work with them to develop a template to guide their interview.
   (1) Questions that an interviewer must not ask (Studer Group, 2010).
      (a) Age.
      (b) Sexual orientation.
      (c) About any health issues (including pregnancy), injuries, disease, or psychiatric problems.
      (d) About drug or alcohol problems.
      (e) Whether the candidate has children, their ages, and child care arrangements.
      (f) If the candidate has ever been arrested.
      (g) Marital status.
      (h) Whether the candidate has ever filed for Workers' Compensation.
      (i) Where the candidate was born or lives.
      (j) Citizenship.
      (k) Religion or church affiliation.
      (l) Political or organizational affiliations.
      (m) Financial status.
      (n) Maiden name.
   (2) Questions regarding the applicant's ability to do this job with or without reasonable accommodations are acceptable (U.S. Equal Opportunity Commission, 2014). Examples of such questions include:
      (a) Can you lift 30 pounds? (If the job duties require lifting that amount of weight.)
      (b) Do you have a driver's license? (If the job requires driving.)
      (c) Are you able to read a computer terminal? (If the job requires use of a computer.)
   (3) If the applicant requires a reasonable accommodation to perform the essential functions of the job for which he or she is being interviewed, this should be discussed.
      (a) It is important at the conclusion of the interview to indicate to the candidate that a disability identified by the candidate will not have an impact on the hiring decision, unless there is a legitimate job requirement that cannot be performed by individuals with certain disabilities even with reasonable accommodations.
      (b) If a human resource department is available, their guidance and assistance with the reasonable accommodation could be beneficial.
   (4) Before making the final decision, assign responsibility for checking references,

doing background checks, and any required drug testing, etc. If available, a human resource department will generally be responsible for these tasks as well as offering the candidate the position and discussing salary and benefits.

d. A new employee's impression of the organization is generally formed in the first 90 days and can impact retention (Studer, 2003). Meeting with the employee at 30 days and again at 90 days will help you identify and remedy any developing issues and help develop the supervisor-employee relationship. Establishing this open channel will encourage future communication, provide feedback which helps improve the workplace, and enhance retention. Examples of questions to ask the new employee include:
   (1) When you were interviewed and hired, I/we presented the organization/ department in a certain way. How closely have we come to meeting your expectations? Please explain.
   (2) When you were interviewed and hired, I/we presented our organization as having a service-oriented culture. Does what we said about our culture accurately represent what you have experienced?
   (3) Do you feel welcome here? Are coworkers willing to assist you?
   (4) What do you like about working here?
   (5) Were there activities or practices at your last job that you think we should adopt here?
   (6) Has anything happened in the last 30 (or 90) days that made you wonder if you had made the right choice about working here?
   (7) Are there any reasons for which you may consider leaving this organization for other employment?
   (8) How am I doing as your supervisor? Do you have enough communication from me regarding your performance or progress?
   (9) What do you know about why we care about the patient's experience?
   (10) Is there any other information I need to know about your first 30 (or 90) days?
   (11) What activities have you heard about or participated in to improve patient and staff safety?
   (12) Have you ever or do you feel you could speak up about something you felt was unsafe?
   (13) Rate each of the following on a scale of 1 to 5:
      (a) I know what is expected of me at work.
      (b) I have the materials and equipment I need to do my work right.
      (c) At work, I have the opportunity to do what I do best every day.
      (d) In the last 7 days, I have received recognition or praise for doing good work.
      (e) My supervisor or someone at work seems to care about me as a person.
      (f) There is someone at work who encourages my development.

D. Staff development.
1. It is important for the leader to proactively engage with employees, constantly evaluate competencies, and offer opportunities for professional development (Studer Group, 2010).
   a. Proactive development. The leader looks ahead at the organization's needs, the learning needs of staff members, and then provides the education and development ahead of time, repeating as needed to assure the staff's success. This is the preferred method of staff development.
   b. Reactive development. Happens after a problem is encountered with unacceptable staff performance, forcing the supervisor to look at the employee's skills. You hope to find this educational need before the lack of needed skills/education has a negative effect on patient outcomes.
2. Preceptors can be used to assist in the development of new staff members and to assure delivery of safe, high-quality care.
   a. "Preceptors are the essential link between what nurses are taught and what they do, and between what nurses know and what they need to know. Having competent preceptors is critical to educating nursing students, transitioning graduate nurses to the professional nursing role, and transitioning experienced nurses to new roles and specialties" (Ulrich, 2012, p. xxv of Introduction).
   b. "A preceptor is an individual with demonstrated competence in a single area who serves as a teacher/coach, leader/influencer, facilitator, evaluator, socialization agent, protector, and role model to develop and validate the competencies of another individual" (Ulrich, 2012, p.xxv-xxvi of Introduction).
   c. Ulrich (2012) describes three common myths about preceptors.
      (1) Myth: *Because you are a good clinical nurse, you will be a good preceptor.* Effective precepting is like a clinical specialty in itself that must be learned by the preceptor.

(2) Myth: *You have to be an expert clinician to become a preceptor.* It is important to be competent in the nursing specialty you are precepting, but sometimes it is a hindrance and frustrating to be much more expert than the nurse you are precepting.
(3) Myth: *Precepting must work around whatever patient assignment is made and whatever is happening on the unit.* Such activity is not precepting. Precepting includes both a competent preceptor and a safe, structured, learning environment.

d. Various roles and relationships in precepting include (Ulrich, 2012):
(1) Teacher/coach role: Common themes important to learning include creating a space for learning, providing concrete illustrations, controlling the opportunities and pace of learning, and allowing some time to reflect on what was taught/learned.
(2) Leader/influencer role: Key aspects of this role include clarifying goals and priorities; freely enlisting others as potential allies to help; identifying the goals and concerns of the preceptee and other team members; determining what is relevant to teach and what is valued by each of the individuals and the organization; taking into account the nature of relationships and how each person wants to interact; and influencing through give and take.
(3) Facilitator role: This includes making assignments to enhance learning and making connections with other clinicians and departments to enable intentionally planned learning opportunities with the goal of achieving a rich positive learning environment for the preceptee.
(4) Evaluator role: Use of criteria-based competencies is helpful as a framework to provide timely, constructive, nonjudgmental criticism to improve or correct specific behaviors, reinforce good performance, and provide suggestions for improvement. A goal is to enhance mutual discussion to change the preceptee's thinking, behavior, and performance.
(5) Socialization agent: "Preceptors facilitate the socialization of preceptees into the organization, into the unit, and even into the nursing shift within a unit by teaching preceptees the norms, the 'sacred cows,' the formal and informal expectations, and the unwritten rules of the game" (Ulrich, 2012, p. 12). This role includes influencing others to be accepting and encouraging to the preceptee as well as facilitating the formation of relationships with other disciplines, including physicians, which is a skill especially important for a new graduate nurse.
(6) Protector: Preceptors protect the safety of patients and of the preceptee by creating a safe learning environment.
(a) This includes interrupting disruptive behavior and lateral/horizontal (nurse on nurse) violence.
(b) Coaching the preceptee on how to speak up regarding bullying or incivility and to involve a manager if necessary.
(7) Role model: Preceptors must practice what they preach and not vary from the steps they have taught the preceptee to accomplish a task.
(a) Although there may be various ways to accomplish a task that result in the same outcome, it is confusing for the learners to see variations in standards of practice and performance.
(b) The role model also takes responsibility to remind other nurses of their role in the education of the preceptee.

e. Preceptors should go through a formal training process before assignment to ensure they will use a disciplined, objective approach and will understand the expectations of both the preceptor role and role of the new employee.
(1) A single preceptor can be assigned, but precepting can also be done successfully using a team approach (with multiple preceptors) and even with cohorted learners (i.e., multiple preceptees).
(2) Keys to success include communication, transparency, and accountability of everyone involved, including the manager and charge nurse (Ulrich, 2012).

f. A written, structured, formal educational process with check-offs by both the preceptor and the new employee is recommended. The time frame for preceptorship averages about 6 to 8 weeks, but the length may vary depending on the position and the individual learner. The learning style of the preceptee must be considered when developing the plan.

g. Each preceptor program must address the following core competencies for all clinicians (Ulrich, 2012).
(1) Providing patient-centered care.
(2) Working in interdisciplinary teams, including teamwork and collaboration.
(3) Employing evidence-based practice.
(4) Applying quality improvement techniques.
(5) Use of informatics.

3. Mentorships. A mentorship program can help extend the support offered to a new employee. It fosters good relationships with other staff members, greatly enhances teamwork, and increases the likelihood that the new staff member will remain on the job (Ulrich, 2012). "Mentoring is a process for the informal transmission of knowledge, social capital, and the psychosocial support perceived by the recipient as relevant to work, career, or professional development; mentoring entails informal communication, usually face-to-face and during a sustained period of time, between a person who is perceived to have greater relevant knowledge, wisdom, or experience (the mentor) and a person who is perceived to have less (the protégé)" (Bozeman & Fenney, 2007, p. 731).
   a. Description of a mentoring program (Ulrich, 2012).
      (1) The new employee can be paired with a mentor for a time period (typically 3 to 6 months) to provide extended clinical and socialization support.
      (2) The mentor should be someone other than the original preceptor to expand the new employee's network of support and also avoid extending the onboarding and orientation budget.
      (3) Monitoring of the mentorship program can be done by the unit manager in collaboration with unit council representatives, if present.
         (a) Establishing a frequent meeting schedule and using formalized feedback tools are helpful in identifying additional learning opportunities.
         (b) Provides the employee with positive feedback on accomplishments.
   b. A mentorship program can be useful in assisting current staff who are struggling with clinical issues or need support with skill/career advancement.
   c. Nurses may want to find their own mentor for guidance with career advancement (Goldmann, 2014). The mentor should help guide rather than supervise and/or give content.
      (1) It is important to find a mentor who is a good fit personally and the relationship between mentor and mentee should feel comfortable.
      (2) The mentor can help facilitate external relationships to establish external credibility and help the mentee build experience for his/her resume.
      (3) The mentee should encourage the mentor to create other kinds of outside opportunities for him/her such as delivering presentations, and serving on editorial boards or committees.
      (4) The mentee has an obligation to make note of the mentor's suggestions, to follow through or let the mentor know why not. It is important that the mentee stop and reflect on his/her experiences and how those feel, and provide feedback to the mentor. The personal advice and opportunities that are acted upon can become the focus of the mentor's written or verbal job recommendations.
   d. It is helpful for the mentee to take on his/her own mentorship role early in his/her career.
      (1) Learning is facilitated by actively assisting others learn.
      (2) As a step toward the mentor role, the individual can work with a more experienced person as a co-mentor.
      (3) Generously giving back to others as a mentor is a great way to enhance personal job satisfaction and boost one's career.
4. Tools such as handouts, intranet modules, and electronic programs can be developed to assure consistency of learning materials. These tools can also be used for annual competency assessments and retraining. Topics of importance to nephrology include:
   a. Infection control.
   b. Medication management.
   c. Safety-related issues. For example, in a dialysis unit, this would include how to test for total chlorine, how to check the conductivity, and the acceptable parameters for these tests.
   d. Equipment use.
   e. Clinical procedures.
   f. Unusual occurrences and emergent situations.
   g. Disaster preparedness. For example, for hemodialysis, this would include the emergency take-off procedures; for transplantation, how to replace a supply of immunosuppressive medications if drugs are lost or destroyed.
   h. Process for patient assessment and care planning.
5. Verification of competency must be done initially and at least annually. Documentation in the personnel record should include a written test(s) and evidence of observations of successful performance(s).
6. Other types of staff development include supporting staff attendance at programs offering continuing education hours, internally (i.e., company sponsored) or externally (e.g., through ANNA, NKF, or ESRD Network meetings).
7. Formal staff evaluations should occur on schedule and be documented. A commonly used schedule

is after the first 30 days of employment, at 90 days, before the 6-month anniversary date, and then annually.

8. Developing employees. Studer discusses the concept of high, middle, and low performers and critical conversations with each group (Studer Group, 2010).
   a. High performers. Focus attention on, recognize, and spend the most time and attention with high performers.
      (1) Characteristics of high performers.
         (a) Trustworthy and proactive about coming to you with solutions.
         (b) Good clinically, and great team players.
         (c) Supportive of everyone including peers, physicians, senior leaders, and the organization.
         (d) Tend to leave the organization/facility if contributions are not rewarded and recognized.
      (2) Conversations with high performers should include:
         (a) Tell them where the organization or facility is headed.
         (b) Thank them for their work using specific examples.
         (c) Tell them why they are important and how they positively contribute to the organization or facility.
         (d) Ask if there is anything you can do for them.
   b. Middle performers. Support and coach middle performers to develop into high performers.
      (1) Characteristics of middle performers.
         (a) Employees you would hire again.
         (b) Generally they aspire to work at higher levels, but may lack experience, skills, or confidence.
         (c) With help they can develop to meet their full potential.
         (d) Dependable and reactive. When a problem is encountered, they are there to help, but they do not necessarily develop or act on a solution.
         (e) Frequently influenced by those around them, so if surrounded by high performers, they will raise their performance level. When surrounded by low performers, they may get dragged into the mindset of that group.
         (f) Need mentoring and clear expectations if they are to reach full potential.
      (2) Middle performer conversations should focus on:
         (a) Reassuring, recruiting, and developing.
         (b) Support by providing specific feedback on what they are doing well.
         (c) Coach by offering one specific opportunity for improvement and the benefit of growing in this area.
         (d) Additional support to reaffirm your confidence in their ability to develop, as well as thanking them for their current contributions.
   c. Low performers. Clarify expectations for improving a skill or behavior with low performers and communicate very real consequences for not making the change.
      (1) Characteristics of low performers.
         (a) Employees you would not rehire.
         (b) Often have a negative attitude and undermine the team.
         (c) May be deficient in clinical skills and/or relationship building.
         (d) Undermine clinical quality and can suck the life out of a team.
         (e) Need to be counseled to move "up or out."
      (2) Low performer conversations should focus on clarifying expectations for improving a skill or behavior and what will happen if the changes are not made.
         (a) Describe the behavior that needs to change. Give specific examples, not generalities, and concentrate on behaviors, not attitudes.
         (b) Evaluate or explain how that behavior affects the performance of the department or facility or outcome for the patient and family. The employee must agree that the problem exists and acknowledge responsibility for his/her behavior. Do not assume that the employee already has knowledge of the problem. The employee must also perceive that the needed change is in his/her best interest.
         (c) Mutually discuss alternative solutions to correct the problem. Don't assume that the employee knows what to do to fix the problem. Face-to-face maximum involvement of the employee in the planning process is a key to success. Get the employee involved, rather than just telling them what to do.
         (d) Mutually agree on the action(s) to be taken to solve problem. Accurately identify the plan for improvement in writing, using specific behavioral examples to clarify.
         (e) Tell the employee the consequences and what will happen if necessary changes are not made.

(f) Set up a timeline for follow-up discussions to identify the progress.
(g) Recognize, acknowledge, and praise any achievement as it occurs and during follow-up.
(h) Document all counseling sessions. Expect the employee to sign and date a work improvement plan. Provide a copy of the plan to the employee. The work improvement plan should include the following:
  i. Description of the problem with specific examples of problematic behavior by the employee.
  ii. Explanation of why this behavior is a problem.
  iii. Mutually agreed-upon plan for improvement.
  iv. Consequences for not making the change.
  v. Follow-up plan with dates and times for meeting.
(i) These conversations may be painful for the low performer, but remember that pain is a motivator and that the employee's poor performance has likely caused pain for others.
(j) It is imperative to follow through on consequences when low performers actions/behaviors do not change. Employees must understand the link between behavioral expectations and consequences. Other employees are counting on the manager to appropriately take follow-up action.

9. Managing organizational change (Studer Group, 2010).
   a. Identify all the stakeholders including all who will be affected by the change.
      (1) What are the barriers to success?
      (2) Who will block the change? How will this be counteracted?
      (3) What are the tough questions that staff will ask? How will they be answered?
      (4) Remember that resistance to change is very personal. Individuals may not resist the change itself, but resist the change being imposed on them.
      (5) Realize that the real challenge of successful change implementation is on the behavioral side.
   b. Identify what ripple effects this change may have in other areas or departments and involve them in the planning.
   c. Identify who will lead the change project.
      (1) Who could be a champion of the change?
      (2) Identify someone who has passion about the change, is respected by others, and has positive influence to deliver the message.
      (3) Make sure whoever leads the project is committed to and believes in it. Individuals cannot lead successfully what they do not believe in!
   d. Carefully plan the change with detailed steps and time schedule.
   e. Before the change, assure there are adequate resources including tools and people power.
   f. Include as many stakeholders as possible from beginning to end, as it builds a sense of ownership, commitment, and accountability for successful implementation.
   g. Provide loud, transparent, effective communication before, during, and after the change.
      (1) Answer the questions: Why the change? Why now?
      (2) Avoid dodging tough questions.
      (3) High visibility and enthusiasm about the change are important. Enthusiasm is contagious!
   h. Celebrate milestones along the way; do not wait until the entire change is implemented to celebrate.
      (1) Show appreciation for any incremental change made; this creates more enthusiasm for the change.
      (2) Create a souvenir of the past to use in celebrations.
   i. After the change, evaluate how it went.
      (1) Is there anything that needs some rework for a better outcome?
      (2) Plan for periodic review of practice to assure there is no sliding back to the old process.

E. Healthy work environment.
   1. All staff members deserve to practice in an environment that is supportive and respectful, as well as where their voices are heard in the efforts to achieve optimal patient outcomes. Patients and families have the right to expect to receive competent, compassionate, high-quality care in a safe, healthy environment (Hanson, 2014). Patient safety hinges on the ability of the healthcare team to work together.
   2. In 2008, the Joint Commission stated, "Safety and quality of patient care is dependent on teamwork, communication, and a collaborative work environment. To assure quality and to promote a culture of safety, healthcare organizations must address the problem of behaviors that threaten the performance of the healthcare team."
   3. In 2005, the American Association of Critical Care Nurses (AACN) identified essential

characteristics of a healthful work environment. Their "Standards for Establishing and Sustaining Healthy Work Environments" include (Hanson, 2014, p. 11):
   a. Skilled communication.
   b. True collaboration.
   c. Effective decision making.
   d. Appropriate staffing.
   e. Meaningful recognition.
   f. Authentic leadership.
4. Ritter (2011) refers to the Nine Principles and Elements of a Healthful Practice/Work Environment, which were developed by the Nursing Organizational Alliance.
   a. Collaborative practice culture (including nurse and physician).
   b. Communication-rich culture.
   c. A culture of accountability.
   d. The presence of adequate numbers of qualified nurses.
   e. The presence of expert, competent, credible, and visible leadership.
   f. Shared decision making at all levels.
   g. The encouragement of professional practice and continued growth and development.
   h. Recognition of the value of nursing's contribution.
   i. Recognition by nurses of their meaningful contribution to practice.
5. An important aspect of a healthy work environment is the development of a culture of safety in which:
   a. Blame is not placed for an error or potential error.
   b. The real and potential systems issues are examined and analyzed.
   c. "A healthy work environment is defined as one that is safe, healing, humane, and respectful of all persons, and fosters the initiative needed for delivery of quality" (Longo & Hain, 2014, p. 194).
6. Inappropriate and aggressive behaviors of healthcare workers toward one another can contribute to the likelihood of making an error, delaying care, and becoming the root cause of adverse events and near misses. Inappropriate behaviors include the following:
   a. Incivility – workplace behaviors that disregard expected norms.
   b. Bullying – persistently picking on or humiliating a coworker or subordinate.
   c. Horizontal violence – harassment between workers of the same rank, such as staff nurse to staff nurse.
   d. Mobbing – one person harassed by a group of workers (Longo & Hain, 2014).
7. Inappropriate behaviors that contribute to an unhealthy work environment.
   a. Examples include intimidation, talking behind someone's back, belittling or criticizing a colleague in front of others, blaming unjustly, treating someone differently, exclusion, social isolation, humiliation, unreasonable demands, verbal abuse, and denied opportunities.
   b. These sorts of behaviors can occur between any categories of healthcare workers; it cannot be assumed that the employee with a higher rank is always the aggressor.
   c. The main impetus for bullying is attaining power – real or perceived.
   d. Adult bullies may in fact be jealous of others.
   e. In cultures where bullying is supported, managers and/or charge nurses may even adopt a bullying management style as a way to accomplish work (Longo & Hain, 2014).
8. Potential patient safety risks and adverse events that can be linked to disruptive behaviors.
   a. Risks include threatened quality of care, medical errors, patient mortality, and near-misses.
   b. Victims of inappropriate behavior can have higher rates of absenteeism, poor work performance, and lower productivity.
   c. Victims may also suffer illnesses including digestive problems, eating disorders, headaches, insomnia, anger, frustration, and psychological distress including self-esteem issues.
   d. The potential for the bullied worker to leave is high, resulting in added fiscal implications for the organization. (Longo & Hain, 2014; Moore et al., 2013).
9. Nurse managers are a key link to enhancing employee retention and ensuring good patient outcomes by ensuring a positive work environment. Managers must demonstrate respect for each employee.
   a. Key practices to promote a healthy work environment include adequate staffing, good orientation, rewards and recognition, nurse-physician collaboration, and autonomy. Encouragement, support of educational growth and development, and opportunities for professional advancement can also improve job satisfaction (Ritter, 2011).
   b. Authentic leadership that encourages openness and consistent sharing of information is an important element. Nurse managers should foster a work setting with a strong sense of community where each person is valued as an important part of the team, where they are empowered as nurses, and where they have access to needed support resources (Moore et al., 2013).

10. Managers must have a strong presence, continuously monitor the work environment, and lead by example to foster the positive work environment.
    a. If bad behavior is ignored, that behavior is essentially condoned.
    b. Leadership must define the nonnegotiable behavioral expectations in writing and require staff commitment to abide by them.
        (1) It is helpful to have a commitment agreement for employees to sign upon hiring.
        (2) These can be reviewed and re-signed annually during employee evaluations.
        (3) In 2014, Tye suggested including the values of compassion, accountability, and respect in behavioral expectations.
        (4) One leadership goal must be to develop a culture of ownership where employees hold themselves accountable for maintaining a positive work environment.
11. Behaviors that help create a nurturing work setting include (Moore et al., 2013):
    a. Using common courtesies.
    b. Avoiding cliques. Instead, be inclusive.
    c. Being respectful.
    d. Being supportive of team members' strengths.
    e. Using open communication.
    f. Guiding new graduates to fit in.
    g. Taking part in decision making for the unit.

F. Patient satisfaction (Studer Group, 2010).
1. A nurse leader making rounds has a powerful effect on the patients' perceptions of care and is a good way to ensure that the care is meeting the quality and satisfaction needs of the patients.
    a. Establishing a rounding discipline.
        (1) Before implementing a rounding routine, obtain buy-in from senior management for time implications by discussing the expected results, which include:
            (a) Better quality outcomes.
            (b) Higher patient perceptions of "good care," resulting in increased market share.
            (c) Enhanced safety and risk reduction.
            (d) Recognition for employees.
            (e) Increased physician and/or provider satisfaction.
            (f) Improves the connection of the nurse leaders with the joy and purpose of their work.
        (2) Work with senior management regarding what to expect and how they can assist with the process.
            (a) Share information from rounding logs.
            (b) "Manage up" through creating a positive impression with supervisory staff by relating good experiences and recognizing staff members who were mentioned favorably by patients.
            (c) Designate "no meeting times of the day" on calendars to institute a routine time for patient rounding.
            (d) Develop and implement a rounding log to keep track of who you saw and what was said.
    b. Getting started – how to round on patients.
        (1) Prior to rounding on patients, check with staff first to let them know you will be rounding and ask if there is anything you should know beforehand about any of the patients.
        (2) Four goals for leader rounding (Studer Group, 2010, p. 116).
            (a) Manage the patient's expectations. For example: "Good morning. I'm Jane Smith, nurse manager of the transplant unit and I stopped by to visit with you. Is this a good time? I want to check in and make sure you are receiving very good care. That is my expectation for all of my patients." The goal is to establish an empathetic, compassionate rapport.
            (b) Service recovery. For example: "How well are we doing in providing your care?" If there are any issues, they can be immediately addressed.
            (c) Harvest recognition (i.e., collect recognition stories) and "manage up" by saying something good about an employee or another person, thus creating a positive impression. For example: "I see that Emma is your nurse today. Emma has more than 20 years of transplant experience. We were very excited a couple of months ago when she was recognized by a national transplant organization with an award for excellence! Is there a staff member who stands out in providing very good care to you? Can you give me an example of that?"
            (d) Manage staff performance by observing for and questioning patients about quality of care and safe environment. For example:
                i. Is patient clean and comfortably positioned?
                ii. Is the call light within reach?
                iii. Does the patient know his/her plan of care for the day?
                iv. Does the patient know the name of his/her nurse?

v. Is the bed or chair-side area clean and free from clutter?

c. At the close of the rounding session, ask the patient: "Is there anything more I can do for you? I have the time."

d. Give daily public recognition to nurses for good patient care and any specific compliments heard during rounds. Say THANK YOU for making it happen!

e. It is very important to hardwire rounding into the schedule.

2. Patient rights and responsibilities.

a. Patients must be advised concerning their rights and responsibilities and have knowledge regarding the grievance procedure.

b. Each hospital or facility must have the grievance policy posted in the patient area.

c. Individuals with kidney failure needing dialysis or transplantation can get help with a grievance from the local ESRD Network or from the state survey agency. Their contact information must also be posted in the patient area (ESRD Network Coordinating Center [NCC], n.d.).

3. Patient Satisfaction Outcome Measurements.

a. Tools used for measurement include:

(1) Consumer Assessment of Healthcare Providers and Systems (CAHPS) surveys are CMS-required measures of the patient's experience of care for both general hospitals and outpatient dialysis facilities. It is important to educate staff regarding the questions asked on the CAHPS surveys to ensure the areas of focus are addressed with patients.

(a) For hospitals, a sample of discharged patients receives the hospital CAHPS survey each month from an outside vendor. The hospital receives a score in the CMS hospital quality management program based on the results of these surveys. Financial penalties can be imposed for poor performance in this area.

(b) In-center hemodialysis (ICH) facilities serving more than 30 adult patients within a year must contract with a vendor to administer the ICH CAHPS. The frequency of the surveys is set by CMS as part of the quality payment criteria. At the time of this writing, the ICH CAHPS survey is a reporting measure. CMS has proposed that the scores for some items on the survey become clinical measures for the 2016 performance period. There would be a risk of low scores resulting in payment reductions.

(2) The Kidney Disease Quality of Life (KDQOL-36) Survey is required to be administered to adult patients on in-center hemodialysis by the CMS ESRD Conditions for Coverage.

(a) Given at 90 days and at least annually to assess physical and mental functioning status.

(b) This survey is generally administered by the social worker, and the results are expected to be used in the patient's plan of care.

(3) Facilities may choose to do other surveys to assess patient satisfaction. These can be either hospital or facility generated and administered, or they can come from and be administered by an outside vendor.

b. Quality assessment and performance improvement (QAPI) actions related to patient satisfaction.

(1) Review patient satisfaction survey results with staff. Post the results and discuss at staff meetings.

(2) Follow up on patient rounding feedback.

(3) Send thank-you notes to staff regarding specific compliments received.

(4) Work on improving problems found by instituting QAPI projects.

(5) Communicate back to patient regarding issue resolution.

(6) Deal with negative patient feedback.

(a) If a minor complaint, apologize, convey that you will follow up, and give feedback.

(b) Service recovery is a formalized approach to effective complaint management or resolution. If the complaint comes with strong emotion and the patient appears to be very upset, it is important to institute the service recovery mode (Studer Group, 2010). This includes a three-step process of recognizing what went wrong, making apologies, and taking action to make amends. It is important to teach front line staff to do service recovery as soon as they see an issue.

i. Acknowledge inconvenience. People are very intolerant of being ignored or having the perception of being ignored.

ii. It is okay to say "I'm sorry" to express regret without necessarily accepting blame.

iii. The "CARE Approach" (Studer Group, 2010, pp 216-217).
C is for Connect. Introduce

yourself, make eye contact, and say, "What is the problem, and how can I make it better for you? Allow patient to vent.

A is for Apologize. No excuses! Confirm that whatever happened is not up to the usual standard of customer care. If the customer has come to you, own the problem. Be careful not to stray into excuses or lay blame. Even if the situation is unavoidable or you feel the customer is unreasonable, you can say you are sorry that the customer is unhappy.

R is for Repair. What would it take to make the customer happy? If the answer is not obvious, ask the question. Sometimes the customer just wants acknowledgment. Ask "What can I do to make it better for you?" Some situations are not within our power to change, but at least an apology can be offered. If possible, give information (not excuses) that will help the patient understand the reasons behind what occurred. Unless there is a compelling contraindication, a corrective action that meets the patient's wishes should be taken.

E is for Exceed. Do not just meet, but instead exceed the customer's expectations. It costs over five times more to recover a customer than it does to get one initially. The economics of service recovery indicates that exceeding expectations is an effort that is well worth the investment (Studer Group, 2010, pp. 216-217). For example, if a patient has been kept waiting and misses his/her bus ride, give him/her a taxi voucher to get home.

(c) How to hardwire a service recovery process with staff.
   i. Create a policy with a clear process and communicate it to all front-line staff.
   ii. Have an easy access notebook, box, or binder with all the tools needed for service recovery, including: cards/envelopes with the organization's logo and with a printed message about how we are sorry not to meet expectations, a tracking log, and an assortment of gifts and vouchers to choose from.
   iii. Encourage and empower staff to use these resources immediately.

c. How to deal with difficult patients who are causing problems in the facility. ESRD Networks provide assistance to both patients and facilities.
   (1) The Networks have a program called "Decreasing Dialysis Patient-Provider Conflict," which can be used in staff training (ESRD Network Coordinating Center [NCC] Homepage, n.d.)
   (2) Network staff can also assist with writing care agreements, which can be an effective way to motivate patients and staff to work together more productively.
   (3) Patients may ask the Network's Medical Review Board to review their complaints regarding facility clinical practice and standards of care.
   (4) In the event an outpatient dialysis facility determines it must discharge or transfer a patient against the patient's wishes, also called an involuntary discharge (IVD) or involuntary transfer, the dialysis facility must engage the ESRD Network for assistance and review.

4. How to individualize patient care for optimal patient satisfaction.
   a. Find out what very good or excellent care means to the patient. Ask each one.
      (1) What is good for one patient might not be what another patient wants.
      (2) Find out what "wows" the patient.
   b. Meaningful care. An interactive team approach, which includes the patient, is needed to develop care plans where the patient's goals, needs, and desires are the drivers for the plan and outcomes (patient-centered care). Leadership's responsibility is to assure there are resources to make this process happen, documentation is completed, and tracking is done to assure the time frames required by CMS are followed.
   c. Organizing support groups and/or coordinating new patient mentors are activities that are helpful to patients and family members. Sharing experiences with others with similar problems is very helpful in learning to navigate the difficult process of coming to terms with chronic kidney disease.
   d. In 2013, CMS and accreditation organizations began to urge healthcare facilities to integrate patients into organizational quality oversight and involve patients in their quality assurance processes. One way to accomplish this would

be to add one or more patients to an action team working on a QAPI project related to direct patient care.

G. Assuring quality of care and improved patient outcomes.
   1. Refer to the QAPI section in this chapter.
   2. Use of the Dialysis Facility Report.
      a. Dialysis facilities receive several electronic reports comparing their outcomes with the outcomes of other dialysis facilities in their state, their Network, and the nation.
      b. The facility supervisor must ensure that the reports are promptly downloaded from the website (http://www.dialysisdata.org) to allow review by the QAPI team for any outcomes where the facility performance falls below the state or national performance.
      c. The draft reports for the Dialysis Facility Report, Dialysis Compare, and the Performance Score Report are posted in July each year.
         (1) Facilities are allowed to comment and question any potential error in the aggregate performance data.
         (2) The final performance score reports must be posted in a patient area within 5 days of being available on that same website near the end of December each year.
   3. Electronic reporting of patient outcome data.
      a. Dialysis facilities are required to submit infection control data to the National Healthcare Safety Network (NHSN) each month to avoid the risk of a payment penalty from the CMS Quality Incentive Program.
         (1) As of 2014, outpatient dialysis facilities receive a score based on the number of blood stream infections per 100 in-center hemodialysis patient months.
         (2) This score will be counted in the Quality Incentive Program (QIP).
         (3) Low scores may result in a payment penalty beginning in the payment year 2016.
      b. CROWNWeb is a web-based data warehouse for information about patients with ESRD. Dialysis facilities are mandated by CMS to enter information about every patient each month.
         (1) This process may take much staff time for Small Dialysis Organizations (SDO) who enter the data manually.
         (2) Large Dialysis Organizations (LDO) are approved by CMS to have the corporate systems submit data in electronic "batches," avoiding manual entries for most of the data.
         (3) The National Renal Administrators Association (NRAA) has made "batch" submission available at a cost for dialysis facilities that use certain brands of electronic medical records.

III. Effective teamwork: staff interaction.

A. Teamwork is critical to the organization.
   1. A team is its own organization with its own dynamics, qualities, and conventions (Templar, 2005).
   2. Teamwork is work done by several individuals with each doing a part but all subordinating personal prominence to the efficiency of the whole (Templar, 2005).
   3. Leaders must seek to build effective, inclusive teams to meet not only patient needs, but also organizational goals, which include:
      a. Staff and patient satisfaction.
      b. Quality outcomes.
      c. Financial stability.
   4. When the team works well together, the outcomes enhance organizational goals. The outcomes include, but are not limited to:
      a. Engaged patients.
      b. Fewer hospitalizations.
      c. Fewer missed treatments.
      d. Effective use of resources and supplies.
      e. Increased patient referrals.

B. In his book, *Leadership: Theory and Practice*, Northouse (2004), describes "team leadership" and gives a functional model of how team leadership works. He states that two very important functions of leadership are to help the group accomplish its task and to keep the group together and functioning.

C. Characteristics of a functional team include:
   1. Clear, elevating goals.
   2. Results-driven structure.
   3. Competent team members.
   4. Unified commitment.
   5. Collaborative climate.
   6. Standards of excellence.
   7. Principled leadership.
   8. External support.

D. Responsibilities and challenges of the chronic kidney disease (CKD) team.
   1. The patient is at the center of the team.
      a. Responsibilities: actively involved in his/her care; commitment to mutually agreed-upon goals.
      b. Challenges: lack of understanding or commitment to the prescribed treatment;

financial limitations, knowledge deficits; and, lack of a functional support system.

2. The nephrologist.
   a. Responsibilities: frequent patient assessments, lead the interdisciplinary team (IDT) in developing the plan of care, oversee medical care, and provide orders for individualized patient care, participate in Quality Assessment Performance Improvement (QAPI) program. If the nephrologist is also the medical director of the facility, further responsibilities include general oversight of the facility, being part of governing body, and being responsible for QAPI.
   b. Challenges: multiple patients at multiple facilities, time constraints, management of patients with many comorbid conditions, expected expertise in water treatment, effective communication with other team members.
3. The advanced practice registered nurse (APRN) or physician assistant (PA).
   a. Responsibilities: in partnership with the physician, oversee patient treatments; participate in the IDT, patient, and staff education; work closely with charge nurse and nurse manager.
   b. Challenges: state limits on practice, effective communication with various levels of staff, variation in expected scope of work.
4. The clinic manager or charge nurse.
   a. Responsibilities: primarily patient care; oversight of unit function; liaison between patient, MD, families, and organizational leadership; active participant in QAPI; part of governing body.
      (1) Clinic manager responsibilities may include personnel, fiscal, and risk management.
      (2) Charge nurse responsibilities may include anemia management, oversee water treatment monitoring, follow up with MD/APRN/PA orders, daily rounding to ensure patient is receiving correct dialysis prescription (e.g., blood flow rate, dialysate concentrate and rate of delivery), and is satisfied with his/her care.
   b. Challenges: staffing issues, time constraints, lack of training for fiscal or risk management responsibilities, patient's lack of understanding or commitment to treatment plan, staff failure to follow policies or standards of care.
5. The licensed practical/vocational nurse (LPN/LVN).
   a. Responsibilities are defined by state practice acts and may include patient care, catheter care, medication administration, oversight of patient care technicians (PCTs).
   b. Challenges: many states limit the practice of the LPN/LVN in an outpatient dialysis facility to that of a PCT, preventing wide use of LPNs/LVNs in many areas of nephrology; practice may also be limited in some hospital settings; requires RN oversight.
6. The registered dietitian.
   a. Responsibilities: nutritional assessments (initial and on-going), coaching related to complex dietary management, management of mineral bone disorder, identification of financial resources related to nutritional needs, required member of the facility's IDT and QAPI team.
   b. Challenges: time restrictions, especially if covering more than one facility or multiple services in a hospital setting; state licensing limitations on practice regarding providing orders and directions for mineral bone disorder management; patient lack of understanding or commitment to treatment plan; support of patients with limited health literacy, language barriers, and/or limited family support.
7. The social worker.
   a. Responsibilities: helping patients adjust to CKD and kidney replacement therapy routine, psychosocial assessments (initial and ongoing), administration of and encouragement of patients to complete Kidney Disease Quality of Life (KDQOL) surveys, assistance with financial resources and insurance coverage issues, follow-up with transplantation referrals, required member of facility IDT and QAPI team.
   b. Challenges: time constraints, especially if covering more than one facility; working with transportation providers; follow-up with transplant evaluations; lack of standardized assessment tools; assistance for patients with limited healthcare coverage; patient lack of understanding or commitment to treatment plan.
8. The patient care technician (PCT).
   a. Responsibilities: delivery of safe and effective patient treatment, maintain certification as required, water treatment monitoring, reinforcement of patient teaching.
   b. Challenges: state-based limits to practice, "over delegation" by inexperienced licensed nurses, achieving required continuing education hours, overlap of patient care duties with the LPN/LVN.
9. The pharmacist.
   a. Responsibilities: in the transplant setting, required by CMS regulations to participate in the multidisciplinary team to assist in

management of medications including immunosuppressives; provide patient education on medications (CMS, 2008c).
   b. Challenges: time constraints, especially if covering multiple services; need to provide complex education within ever-shortening hospital stays; collaboration with the team to ensure education from all parties is planned and congruent.

E. The team is formed as each member supports the others to improve the function of the team as a whole. The expected outcome of a well-functioning team is quality patient care.
   1. Many of the above challenges are faced by teams in different areas of nephrology. One of the most effective ways to overcome these challenges is by maintaining excellent leadership and communication skills.
   2. Every team should have goals and a plan to accomplish those goals. However, as Colin Powell said, "…it is people who get things done…." Powell adhered to two interrelated premises: one, people are competent; and two, every task is important (Harari, 2002). The way these premises are communicated to the team will determine the team's success or failure in accomplishing the goal.
   3. Facilitate effective teamwork and collaboration. The main goal is to optimize the timely and effective use of information, skills, and resources by teams of healthcare providers for the purpose of enhancing the quality and safety of patient care (Agency for Healthcare Research and Quality [AHRQ], 2008). This can be achieved a number of ways, but some required key elements include:
      a. Structure: compose the team, making sure the right people are working together.
      b. Leadership: facilitate optimal team performance, coordination of team efforts, and provision of necessary resources.
      c. Awareness: clear understanding of goals, team responsibilities, situational environment assessment, and progress toward achieving the goals.
      d. Skills: ability of the team to continually gather and assess information; mutual support and timely feedback and backup; open and ongoing communication.
      e. A summary of the above can be broken down to the following:
         Right information – *provided to the*
         right person(s) – *at the*
         right time – *results in the*
         right actions.
   4. Measuring team effectiveness.
      a. Can be difficult to achieve since there are few tools that reliably measure behaviors affecting team functioning.
      b. However, the Team Functioning Assessment Tool (TAFT) is one tool that has been shown to measure clinical planning, executive tasks, and team relations that are important elements of effective multidisciplinary healthcare team functioning (Sutton et al., 2011).
      c. Consider the following when evaluating the effectiveness of a team:
         (1) Perception of elements in the environment.
         (2) Clinical interpretation.
         (3) Case management.
         (4) Identification and utilization of resources.
         (5) Execution of meetings.
         (6) Leadership.
         (7) Innovation.
         (8) Appropriate communication.
         (9) Participative information exchange.
         (10) Appropriate use of authority and assertiveness.
         (11) Consideration of others.

IV. Communication.

A. Definition: the act or process of using words, sounds, signs, or behaviors to express or exchange information or to express your ideas, thoughts, feelings, etc., to someone else (Webster's Third New International Dictionary, 1993).

B. Communication requires a sender, a receiver, and a message. There are six steps in the communication process (Cherie & Gebrekidan, 2005).
   1. Ideation: the message to be conveyed.
   2. Encoding: the way the message is conveyed.
   3. Transmission: conveying the actual message.
   4. Receiving: listening to the message.
   5. Decoding: the receiver's understanding of the message.
   6. Response: conveys the understanding of the message.

C. Methods of communication.
   1. Verbal: words used to convey the message.
      a. Words are individually interpreted.
      b. It is possible to hear the same words but understand the meaning differently.
   2. Nonverbal: gestures, postures, tone of voice, facial expressions, etc. Nonverbal cues can contradict or reinforce the verbal communication.
   3. Electronic: communicating using various electronic means (e.g., email, text, Twitter).
      a. Electronic messages allow almost instant communication between multiple parties.
         (1) It is risky is to assume that everyone received, opened, read, and understood the message.

      (2) Electronic messages may be misinterpreted as they lack inflection and tone of voice as well as visual cues available when individuals are face-to-face.
   b. Care is required to prevent the transfer of personal health information via unsecure electronic systems.

D. Variables that influence the communication process (Weinfield & Donahue, 1989).
   1. No two people see things exactly the same way.
   2. Self-image affects how the world is seen.
   3. Past experiences are influential.
   4. Personal judgment and impressions of another person affect relationships.
   5. Values affect perceptions.
   6. Perceptions vary with time.
   7. Individuals see what they want to see.
   8. The propensity is to see things largely as they have been seen before.
   9. Emotions color what is seen.
   10. There is an inclination to simplify or complicate what is not understood.
   11. The first and last things in a series are remembered the best.
   12. New experiences lead to new ways of perceiving.

E. Basics of good communication (Cherie & Gebrekidan, 2005).
   1. Clarify ideas before communicating to others.
   2. Consider the setting, both physical and psychological.
   3. Consult with others when necessary to be objective.
   4. Be mindful of overtones when delivering a message.
   5. Take the opportunity to convey something that helps, values, or praises the receiver.
   6. Follow up on communications.
   7. Insure actions support communication.
   8. Be an active listener.
   9. Give credit for the contributions of others when it is deserved.
   10. Be assertive when expressing views.

F. Communication styles.
   1. Nonassertive/passive or submissive.
      a. The person does not question or confront the message at the time of delivery; yet later, complains or blames others who have no ability to affect the decision.
      b. "Poor me" types describe themselves as a victim.
      c. Low self-esteem, unwillingness to risk disapproval with unmet needs.
      d. Expects disappointment and rejection.
   2. Aggressive.
      a. Hostile, combative, energetic, and enterprising.
      b. One-way conversations, especially with subordinates.
      c. Appears rude and not open to hearing from others.
      d. Makes quick decisions without much or any input from staff or peers.
      e. Aggressive behavior may hide a sense of insecurity or lack of confidence.
      f. Aggressive behavior by managers does not support the team approach to work.
      g. Staff work in fear of making a mistake rather than with motivation to do things right.
      h. Manipulative and overly direct.
      i. Emotional outbursts common.
   3. Assertive: the preferred style. Assertive communication skills encompass:
      a. Ownership of one's own feelings.
      b. Use of "I" statements (not YOU) and use of objective statements that do not judge another person.
      c. Make a DEAL (Weinfield & Donohue, 1989, p. 109).
         (1) D = Describe one's own emotions and other's behavior.
         (2) E = Express feelings as a result of behavior; place no blame.
         (3) A = Ask for a specific change.
         (4) L = List consequences if necessary.
      d. Positive body language (nonverbal communication).
         (1) Face the listener.
         (2) Use hand gestures.
         (3) Let facial expressions support the assertive message.
         (4) Speak firmly and audibly.
         (5) Maintain good eye contact.
         (6) Sit or stand comfortably with shoulders back and relaxed.
         (7) Look confident.
         (8) Avoid nervous mannerisms.
         (9) Do not negate a serious message by smiling.
      e. Responses to a request.
         (1) Answer promptly and to the point.
         (2) Request more time or information if necessary.
         (3) If a request seems unreasonable, say so.
         (4) Don't overexplain.
         (5) Don't apologize for a decision.
      f. Characteristics of appropriate listening habits.
         (1) Listen with eyes as well as ears.
         (2) Listen between the lines.
         (3) Try to anticipate but remain flexible.
         (4) Pick out key words.
         (5) Weigh what is said versus what you know.
         (6) Constantly analyze.

(7) Weigh evidence by questioning it.
(8) Categorize important points.
(9) Screen out the irrelevant.
(10) Stay alert.

g. Inappropriate listening habits.
(1) Calling the subject uninteresting.
(2) Criticizing the speaker's delivery.
(3) Getting overstimulated by a single point or word.
(4) Listening only for facts.
(5) Trying to outline or take notes on everything.
(6) Faking attention to the speaker.
(7) Tolerating or creating distractions.
(8) Avoiding difficult material.
(9) Allowing emotion-laden words to antagonize.
(10) Wasting the advantage point.

G. Barriers to communication: Obstacles that can prevent the message from being delivered or understood.
1. Criticizing.
2. Name-calling.
3. Diagnosing.
4. Ordering.
5. Threatening.
6. Moralizing.
7. Excessive/inappropriate questioning.
8. Advising.
9. Diverting.
10. Logical argument.
11. Reassuring.
12. If you do not say anything, you condone it.
13. Errors of omission. Do not assume you understand; always validate assumptions.

V. Electronic health records (EHR).

A. Most healthcare institutions have adopted or are moving quickly toward adopting electronic health records (EHR).
1. Having access to patient health information in an electronic format allows the provider to build in monitoring and alerts for an individual patient, for a specific group of patients, or even for a broad group that might stretch across the nation.
2. The government, under the Medicare program, made available financial incentives to certain organizations (e.g., hospitals, physicians' office practices) for using EHR systems to improve patient care.
a. The term *meaningful use* has been coined to describe the electronic criteria, capabilities and processes required to achieve and prove effective use of an electronic record system.
b. To achieve *meaningful use* and avoid financial penalties in the future, providers and organizations must follow a prescribed set of criteria that serve as a roadmap for effective use of EHR and provide documentation of compliance with these requirements.

B. The value of electronic healthcare documentation.
1. Standardized language and definitions.
2. Legible.
3. Visual alerts for safety and quality can be programmed to be automatic.
4. Built-in reminders.
a. Documentation requirements for reimbursement.
b. Performing ordered activities.
c. Timelines for assessments.
d. Timelines for medication administration.
5. Ability to quickly and easily see the documentation of others.
6. Dynamic with easy links to various parts of the record.
7. Easily searched for evaluation of continuity of care and quality assurance activities.
8. Ability to do bedside verification of the patient identification with an ordered medication prior to administration of medications, decreasing the risk of errors and improving patient safety.
9. Built-in warnings for allergies and potential dangerous interactions with other medications.

C. Considerations when using and/or designing an electronic documentation system.
1. Involve the end users in the design.
2. The documentation must tell the story of the patient. This may require some periodic entry of freehand notes in addition to clickable queries.
3. Charting of assessment by exception is acceptable and saves time.
a. This method of charting focuses time and efforts on findings that are outside of normal limits that need to be addressed in the plan of care.
b. One quick click can be made for routine assessments that are within normal limits (WNL). The established normal limits need to be available for reference.
4. Do not overbuild queries to the point it makes the system tedious and time consuming for end users. Involve the end-users in the design of the queries and make sure the queries follow their actual workflow.
5. Fields can be made "mandatory" if the information that is required for that field must be captured for important quality measures or reimbursement. Making too many fields mandatory ties up completion of the document and can be very frustrating to staff.

6. Use of a nurse informatics specialist is of great benefit to organizations that build the majority of their own queries and assessments within the framework of a large EHR system.

D. Choosing a system for EHR.
   1. Integrated systems do not need interfaces for one part of the system to talk to another part.
      a. Generally easier and less expensive to operate in the long run.
      b. Some vendors of integrated systems: Enterprise EHR Vendors, Allscripts, Cerner, Epic, McKesson, Meditech, and Siemons.
   2. Interfaced systems are composed of one type of system for one function and another type of system for a different function. This may seem a smart choice when looking only at the features of each individual system.
      a. It can be difficult and costly to get different computer systems to talk back and forth between one another by the use of interfaces.
      b. When one system needs upgrading, the interfaces also need upgrading. This requires a considerable amount of work and testing to assure the systems will continue to work together.
   3. It would behoove a small dialysis facility to choose an EHR system that is capable of interfacing with the National Renal Administrators Association's (NRAA's) Health Information Exchange (HIE) interface to upload data to CROWNWeb. Go to http://www.nraa.org to see the current list of certified vendors.

E. Transferring records and the Health Insurance Portability and Accountability Act (HIPAA).
   1. As with any healthcare record, strict compliance with HIPAA rules must be met for electronic transfer of records.
   2. Certain information may be electronically transferred to government agencies without the permission of the patient.
      a. This includes the reporting of certain communicable diseases and immunizations given.
      b. Recognize that information relating to immunizations transferred electronically to a government agency may not be transferred subsequently from there to a third party (such as to a school) without authorization by the patient.

VI. Collaboration with the ESRD Network (ESRD NCC, 2014).

A. Eighteen ESRD Network Organizations work under contract to CMS and serve as liaisons between the federal government and the providers of ESRD services.
   1. The number and concentration of ESRD beneficiaries in each geographic area determine the composition of each Network, with some Networks representing one state, some representing multiple states, and one state (California) being split between two Networks.
   2. The End-Stage Renal Disease (ESRD) Network Coordinating Center (NCC) provides centralized coordination and support for the ESRD Network Program. The NCC's primary responsibilities include:
      a. Collection, maintenance, and distribution of ESRD information.
      b. Coordination of national activities, including training initiatives.
      c. Facilitation of special projects and administrative support services.

B. ESRD Networks: responsibilities and facility implications.
   1. Quality oversight of the care received by patients with CKD stage 5.
      a. Patient outcome quality goals.
         (1) Developed by each Network's medical review board.
         (2) Monitored by the Network's quality improvement staff members.
      b. Facilities may be required to participate in Network-based quality improvement projects if the facility consistently fails to meet the Network's standards or goals.
   2. Collection and analysis of data to administer the national Medicare ESRD program. For example:
      a. Dialysis facilities routinely submit monthly data via CROWNWeb.
      b. Subsequently, facilities may be asked to submit additional data at various times for Network-specific quality improvement projects.
   3. Provision of technical assistance to the providers and to patients in areas related to ESRD. As an example, the Network can provide oversight and assistance to both patients and facilities in cases of potential involuntary discharge or transfer of a patient or a patient grievance.

C. Each Network maintains a website with information for patients, transplant programs, and dialysis facilities. To locate the website for a particular ESRD Network, go to http://www.esrdnetworks.org, and click on the state of interest to be directed to the appropriate ESRD Network.

D. Consultation with network staff is available to provide technical assistance upon request. Some of the services available include:
   1. Posts of educational events.

2. Provision of speakers for educational events.
3. Links to documents regarding the ESRD Conditions of Coverage.
4. Information on the CMS's Quality Incentive Program (QIP).
5. Quality Improvement tools on a variety of topics.
6. Skilled nursing facility educational links.
7. Social services and vocational rehabilitation information.
8. News bulletins and FDA alerts.
9. Job listings.
10. CROWNWeb information and assistance.
11. Information on transplant programs.
12. "Fistula First" tools and sample procedures.
13. Email bulletins.
14. Facility lists and contact information.
15. Summary statistics.
16. Data forms.
17. Assistance in managing challenging patient situations and involuntary discharge/transfer.
    a. Networks provide a "Decreasing Dialysis Patient Provider Conflict" Toolkit.
    b. Includes a variety of vignettes and guidance in constructive ways of interacting with patients and staff.
18. Information related to the Dialysis Facility Reports.
19. Patient- and family-centered care resources.
20. Disaster resources.

E. Examples of ESRD Network resources for patients.
1. Networks provide assistance with patient complaints or grievances to include immediate advocacy and quality of care review. The Network may:
    a. Facilitate communication when there is a problem between a patient and a provider or practitioner.
    b. Investigate a patient complaint, requesting that the facility provide information and patient and facility administrative records as needed to resolve the issue.
    c. As charged by CMS, be an advocate for the patient in any grievance and in the event of an allegation of an access to care issue (CMS, n.d.).
2. Consumer newsletters, which may include personal stories from patients with CKD.
3. Emergency preparedness and response, including providing information regarding which facilities are open during or after a natural disaster or other emergency.
4. Patient education materials on a variety of topics such as infection control, vaccinations, depression, quality of life, advance care planning, vascular access choices, transplant selection criteria, and self-care information.
5. Medicare resources.
6. Patient advisory committee information.
7. Vocational rehabilitation information.

VII. Economics.

A. Brief history of ESRD reimbursement. For more detail, go to http://www.annanurse.org/download/reference/health/esrdReimbursementFactSheet.pdf
1. Dialysis was initially available only as a "rescue" treatment.
    a. It was for patients who were thought to be able to recover their kidney function after an acute kidney injury.
    b. Once a vascular access method was developed, allowing repeated use of the same blood vessels for dialysis, Congress was lobbied to provide funding sufficient to support chronic dialysis.
2. The Social Security (SS) Amendments of 1972. https://www.govtrack.us/congress/bills/92/hr1/text
    a. Extended Medicare coverage to individuals less than 65 years of age with ESRD if he/she qualified for SS.
    b. Payment for dialysis was limited to $138 per treatment.
3. ESRD Program Amendments, 1978.
    a. Included provisions to encourage home dialysis.
    b. Extended transplant coverage, including immunosuppressive medications, to 36 months posttransplant.
4. Omnibus Reconciliation Act (OBRA), 1981. https://www.govtrack.us/congress/bills/97/hr3982
    a. Established a single "composite" rate.
        (1) The composite rate payment included equipment, supplies, personnel, and overhead to provide dialysis.
        (2) Medications, other than those required to accomplish dialysis (e.g., heparin, saline, lidocaine) were not included.
        (3) Payment for physicians was not included.
    b. Average payment was $123 per treatment.
5. Medicare Modernization Act (MMA), 2003. https://www.govtrack.us/congress/bills/108/hr1
    a. Composite rate was increased by 1.5%.
    b. Payment for drugs was based on the Average Sales Price (ASP) +6%.
    c. Provided for the drug "add-on" payment to be adjusted annually.
    d. Required Health & Human Services to report on a fully bundled prospective payment system (PPS).
        (1) Fully bundled rate would include items covered under the composite rate plus medications related to CKD stage 5 (e.g., erythropoiesis-stimulating agents [ESA], iron, vitamin D, phosphate binders).
        (2) Would not include physician payment.

6. Medicare Improvements for Patients and Providers Act (MIPPA) of 2008. http://www.gpo.gov/fdsys/pkg/PLAW-110publ275/pdf/PLAW-110publ275.pdf
   a. Required a PPS with a bundled rate to include an annual update.
      (1) PPS implemented in 2011.
      (2) Set a base bundled rate of $230 per treatment.
   b. The Centers for Medicare & Medicaid Services (CMS) was required to establish a Quality Improvement Program (QIP). The QIP would impose a financial penalty of up to 2% of the total Medicare payment to an ESRD facility based on the performance score of that facility using the CMS-specified patient outcome measures.
7. American Taxpayers Relief Act (ATRA) of 2012. https://www.govtrack.us/congress/bills/112/hr8/text
   a. Because of changes in the use of drugs and biologicals (e.g., ESAs, iron, vitamin D) as a result of the PPS, CMS was required to recalculate the bundled payment for payment year (PY) 2014.
   b. Delayed inclusion of oral drugs (e.g., phosphate binders) into the bundle until 2016.
8. Final Rule for ESRD PPS for PY 2016 (CMS, 2013b).
   a. Included a cut to the bundled rate to be phased in over 3 to 4 years.
   b. Almost all of the PPS cut for PY 2014 was offset by omitting the scheduled increases in the bundled rate.
9. Protecting Access to Medicare Act (PAMA) of 2014. http://www.gpo.gov/fdsys/pkg/BILLS-113hr4302enr/pdf/BILLS-113hr4302enr.pdf
   a. Limited the ATRA required cuts to the bundled rate.
   b. Postponed inclusion of oral drugs (e.g., phosphate binders) into the bundle until 2024.
10. Future changes to the ESRD PPS and QIP.
   a. CMS is required to publish a Notice of Proposed Rulemaking (NPRM) each year to propose changes to the PPS and QIP.
      (1) The NPRM is generally published in early July each year with a 60-day comment period.
      (2) Public comments, including comments from ANNA, have influenced the Final Rule, which is required to be published by November 1 each year.
   b. ANNA is actively involved in advocating for nephrology nurses and people with kidney disease. For up-to-date information on proposed and final rules for the PPS and QIP visit http://www.annanurse.org.

B. Quality Incentive Program (QIP) (CMS, 2014). http://www.cms.gov/Medicare/Quality-Initiatives-Patient-Assessment-Instruments/ESRDQIP/
   1. CMS goals for ESRD QIP measures are meant to promote high-quality care and to strengthen the goals of the National Quality Strategy, while protecting patients from potential cuts to services based on changes to the method of payment.
      a. The PPS made medications a cost center rather than a revenue producer.
      b. The potential exists for doses of expensive medications to be reduced to cut costs, with negative effects on patient outcomes, such as anemia management.
   2. MIPPA required that CMS use National Quality Forum (NQF) endorsed measures when available.
      a. The law allowed CMS to add measures if NQF endorsed measures do not exist or are not sufficient for the topic area.
      b. The law requires inclusion of measures on anemia management and dialysis adequacy. MIPPA requires the measures on "anemia management reflect the labeling approved by the Food and Drugs Administration for such management" (MIPPA, 2008).
   3. The QIP includes two kinds of measures.
      a. Reporting measures: the facility is required to report certain information and receives a score based on whether or not the information was reported. In some instances, a percentage (of information to be reported) may apply; in other instances, the facility must attest that the required action was taken.
         (1) Examples of reporting measures that have been used in the QIP include:
            (a) Administration of the In-Center Hemodialysis Consumer Assessment of Healthcare Professionals and Systems (ICH-CAHPS) survey.
            (b) Serum phosphorus levels.
      b. Clinical measures: the facility is given a performance score based on the percentage of eligible patients who meet or exceed the goal for a specified outcome. Examples of clinical measures that have been used in the QIP include:
         (1) Percentage of adult patients on hemodialysis with an adequacy measure equal to or greater than 1.2.
         (2) Percentage of patients on ESA with hemoglobin level above 12 g/dL.
         (3) Percentage of patients using a central venous catheter as dialysis vascular access for greater than 90 days.
         (4) Percentage of blood stream infections in patients per 100 patient months. This clinical measure applies to patients on in-center hemodialysis.

c. For more information and specifications of the current QIP measures, visit http://www.dialysisdata.org

Section D
Quality Assurance and Performance Improvement
Bonnie B. Greenspan

I. The purpose of Quality Assessment and Performance Improvement (QAPI).

A. **Monitor** safety and effectiveness of facility processes and strategies.

B. **Recognize** opportunities for improvement by comparison to community standards and facility trends.

C. **Address** those opportunities with timely and objectively effective action.

D. For outpatient dialysis facilities, effective QAPI allows:
1. Compliance with the federal mandate to achieve:
   a. Measurable improvement in health outcomes.
   b. Reduction of medical errors.
2. Effective usage of indicators or performance measures associated with improved health outcomes and with the identification and reduction of medical errors (CMS, 2008b).

II. MONITORING readiness, effectiveness, and safety: the program's structure and scope. The process requires team commitment, discipline, focus, coordination, and time in order to achieve purposes.

A. Structure.
1. QAPI team composition includes mandatory participation of interdisciplinary members. For outpatient dialysis, this includes the Medical Director, RN, MSW, RD (CMS, 2008b). Additional participation by biomedical and direct care personnel as well as experts (such as patients) is incorporated as appropriate to drive desired performance.
2. Meetings are regularly scheduled (and held) and:
   a. Allow sufficient time for meaningful review of full scope.
   b. Establish frequency of review for specific elements based on the facility's needs and priorities.
   c. Use community standards as benchmarks and thresholds.
   d. May use a variety of presentation and problem identification methods, including virtual participation, but must result in accountable plans for action where needed.

B. Scope.
1. The scope of the facility QAPI program includes monitoring the readiness, effectiveness, and safety for each program offered by the facility. For example, for kidney transplant, this would include pretransplant, peritransplant, and posttransplant quality indicators. For dialysis, this would include quality indicators for all modalities offered (e.g., in-center, nocturnal, home hemodialysis, PD).
2. Poor outcomes or recurring errors alert the team to failures of effectiveness. However, attentiveness to facility readiness through testing, tracking, and auditing enables identification and remediation of risks before impact.
3. Basic monitoring is federally mandated for both dialysis and transplant programs, but facility-specific factors may indicate a need for more intense review.
4. Monitoring requires reporting of the findings to the QAPI team with timeliness appropriate to the alert level, as well as targeted response to identified risks.

C. Monitoring for READINESS applies to both personnel and equipment.
1. Monitoring equipment for readiness must include, but is not limited to:
   a. For hemodialysis, water, and dialysate quality (separate review of in-center and home results).
      (1) Chemical analysis of product water.
      (2) Monthly water and dialysate microbial content (bacteria and endotoxin).
      (3) Total chlorine testing.
      (4) Reverse osmosis system daily monitoring.
   b. Dialysis equipment repair and maintenance.
   c. Physical plant safety.
   d. Furnishings and small equipment intact and appropriate for repeated disinfection.
2. Monitoring of personnel readiness must include, but is not limited to:
   a. Appointments and credentials for medical staff.
   b. Appropriate licensure, certification, and qualifications for all staff.
   c. Annual competence testing to verify:
      (1) Understanding of expectations of position and capability to meet expectations.
      (2) Focused evaluation of emergency preparedness and infection control practices.
   d. Appropriate staff health screenings and immunizations.
   e. Performance audits for key processes.

f. Review and reinforcement or replacement of facility policies and procedures.
g. Staff turnover.
h. Ongoing evaluation of adequacy of number and skillset of the staff to meet patient safety needs.

D. Monitoring of EFFECTIVENESS applies to the achievement of therapeutic goals of care.
1. Monitoring effectiveness of outcomes includes trending the percentage of patients achieving facility goals which meet, at a minimum, the community standard level. For outpatient dialysis, this includes at least the following indicators (CMS, 2008b):
a. Mortality.
b. Hospitalizations.
c. Choice of modality.
d. Dialysis access (HD, PD) selection and status.
e. Adequacy.
f. Anemia.
g. Blood pressure.
h. Fluid management.
i. Nutritional status.
j. Mineral and bone management.
k. Infections.
l. Immunizations.
m. Health outcomes: physical and mental functioning.
2. Measures Assessment Tool (MAT).
a. The MAT is a list of standards developed and maintained by CMS and is considered part of the Conditions for Coverage for ESRD.
b. The MAT lists goals for a number of critical measures that represent evidence-based community consensus standards.
c. The listing references the Condition for Coverage which mandates monitoring and addressing the measure, current minimum standard or target range, and the source authority for the standard for that measure.
d. Developed to assist surveyors in facility review.
e. The MAT is useful and available to all members of the kidney community as well as the general public.
f. The MAT is frequently updated to stay current with community practice standards. Therefore, a copy is not included in this chapter.
g. The URL is long and may change for an individual tool. The simplest way to access the current MAT is to Google the terms "CMS ESRD survey tools."
(1) Choose the link to Dialysis Centers for Medicare & Medicaid Services.
(2) Scroll down to link for the Measures Assessment Tool which may be included in "Surveyor Laminates."
(3) If viewing this information on an electronic reader, this is the link: http://www.cms.gov/Medicare/Provider-Enrollment-and-Certification/GuidanceforLawsAndRegulations/Dialysis.html
(4) A list of all V-tags for the Conditions for Coverage as well as the full regulations and interpretive guidance can be found at the same website.

E. Monitoring SAFETY applies to a systematic effort to obtain all input possible to identify risks and errors as the first step in reducing or eliminating them.
1. Patient satisfaction and perception of care is an integral part of this assessment.
2. Risk reporting is encouraged and expected, analyzed and never punished.
3. Error reporting is rigorous, analyzed in a nonsuperficial way and includes, at a minimum reportables, medical errors, adverse occurrences, clinical variances, and "near misses."
a. The University of Texas studied the use of the term "good catches" along with other leadership support efforts to reduce the negative connotation and increase the recognition of the importance of reporting of what they previously called "near misses."
b. Initial results showed increased reporting. Later expansion of the concept into a baseball-themed competition for reporting and addressing "good catches" produced dramatic increases and wide participation in reporting (Mick et al., 2007).
4. An error is defined by the Institute of Medicine as "the failure of a planned action to be completed as intended or the use of a wrong plan to achieve an aim" (Kohn et al., 2000). The following list represents the minimum elements required by CMS to be reported/tracked (CMS, 2008b).
a. Cardiac arrest at facility or during home treatment.
b. Deaths during dialysis.
c. Errors in dialysis prescription delivery.
d. Medication errors, omissions, adverse reactions.
e. Use of an incorrect dialyzer (new or reprocessed).
f. Blood loss > 100 cc.
g. Total chlorine or other contaminant breakthrough.
h. Machine malfunction with treatment interruption.
i. Unplanned patient transfers by ambulance.
j. Patient transfers to hospital from dialysis.
k. Patient falls.
l. Vascular access infiltration.
m. Intradialytic symptoms.
n. Hypotension with loss of consciousness.

o. Chest pain.
p. Severe cramping.
q. Nausea/vomiting.
r. Staff incidents.
(1) Needle sticks.
(2) Nonadherence to procedures.
(3) Patient abuse or disrespect.
(4) Patient and staff injuries.

5. Error reporting.
a. Reporting of errors is the critical first step in understanding and eliminating system vulnerabilities.
b. The report of the Office of the Inspector General (January 2012), "Hospital Incident Reporting Systems Do Not Capture Most Patient Harm," indicated that only 14% of medical errors are reported. This low reporting was attributed in part to misperceptions by staff of what constitutes patient harm or requires reporting (Levinson, 2012).
c. The availability of a list of "must report" occurrences serves to remind staff that input of this information is crucial to system improvement. However, a simple nonjudgmental rule is more user-friendly and may result in more comprehensive reporting. For example, "When a treatment is not delivered as ordered, review for possible report when results are not as desired."
d. Management should both encourage and expect reporting. The ability to speak up about serious concerns (e.g., poor performance, poor teamwork, disrespect) leads to positive outcomes for patients, the setting, and the staff (Maxfield et al., 2005, p. 7).
e. Use of reporting to identify and reduce vulnerabilities increases safety and reinforces the safety system. Failure to review and act upon reports reinforces underreporting.

III. RECOGNIZING opportunities for improvement.

A. Considerations include the establishment of goals and thresholds.
1. Determine whether current strategies are effective or require revision.
2. Drive appropriate intensity of response.

B. Facility QAPI goals must meet or exceed community standards (e.g., KDOQI, AAMI, ANNA).
1. Some of the community standards can be found on the CMS MAT: http://www.cms.gov/Medicare/Provider-Enrollment-and-Certification/GuidanceforLawsAndRegulations/Dialysis.html
2. Intermediate short-term goals may be useful in clarifying expectations for an acceptable rate of progress in improvement or the response to specific interventions when multiple steps are required.

C. Thresholds should allow action to be triggered (or elevated in priority) in areas previously assessed as well controlled.
1. Thresholds are used to establish alert levels for indicators that drop below (or rise above, in the case of error thresholds) the current expected level.
2. Use of thresholds is expected when a performance improvement process has achieved the desired goal. This assures ongoing effectiveness of the effort over time.
3. Thresholds are also helpful in drawing attention to a need for increased prioritization when a stable indicator begins to trend in an undesired direction. This could lead to more frequent reviews on the facility QAPI calendar.

D. Recognizing a need for revision, improved implementation, or intensification of facility strategies will typically lead to improvement in achievement of goals or reduction in errors.

E. The initial response phase may include:
1. Collection of additional data.
2. Breakdown of existing improvement opportunities into smaller subsets.
a. For example: 50% of facility patients have lab values out of range for phosphorous control. Strategy would include individual lab reviews for all patients, with subgroups targeted for more intense focus, such as:
(1) A patient's phosphorous level suddenly rises over 5.5 mg/dL (milligrams per deciliter) who may be facing new obstacles or burnout on the effort of adherence.
(2) Patients whose current phosphorous is greater than a threshold such as 6.5 mg/dL or 7 mg/dL because of their increased risk.
(3) Patients who are close to target and who may benefit from broad staff involvement and encouragement.
(4) Patients with a 3-month upward trend; attempt to identify the cause and stop the trajectory.
b. Segmenting the problem allows targeted strategies and enables the development of goals rather than wishes.
3. A literature review.
4. A disciplined cause analysis (see cause analysis later in this section).
5. Use of peer mentors or consultation.

F. Potential obstacles to effective responses.
1. Reluctance to report potential or actual problem.
2. Premature assumption of cause or "artifact." If the patient population within a facility has a high percentage of persons who are indigent, elderly, with many comorbidities, etc., then strategies should be adopted to target that particular patient population rather than accepting poor outcomes.
3. Repeated "give it another month" or "continue current plan" approach.
4. Failure to include relevant people (e.g., direct care staff, patients) in understanding problems and potential solutions.
5. Pat, generic responses such as "give in-service" or "repeat routine education" are unlikely to drive change.
   a. Although writing a policy or conducting an in-service seems an appropriate response to failure of staff to "do what they are supposed to," these measures alone are weak solutions to persistent problems.
   b. Simplification and standardization have a greater likelihood of success when automation or engineering is not called for or possible.
   c. Figure 1.7 illustrates the comparative effectiveness of various protective strategies that may be employed to enhance patient safety (Veteran's Administration, n.d.).

G. Seized opportunities for improvement.
1. The dialysis industry has responded to safety challenges with engineering responses from the initiation of air detectors, to the regulation of saline prime volume, and a wide array of hard alarms and visual indicators.
2. In infection control and team communication, safety imperatives depend upon consistent human adherence to procedural expectation. The combination of support, expectation, and consequence required to achieve that adherence is not likely to be accomplished by a policy or in-service alone.

IV. Considerations in ADDRESSING opportunities for improvement.

A. Once an error or an outcome below community standard is identified, or an outcome is above that standard but represents a drop in an individual facility's performance, the most challenging element of QAPI occurs: identifying and eliminating the cause(s) of underperformance. The cause(s) are most often multifaceted.

B. While a cause can sometimes be immediately identified and eliminated, more often the cause is complex and includes a breach in more than one of the layers of protection established for the unit.

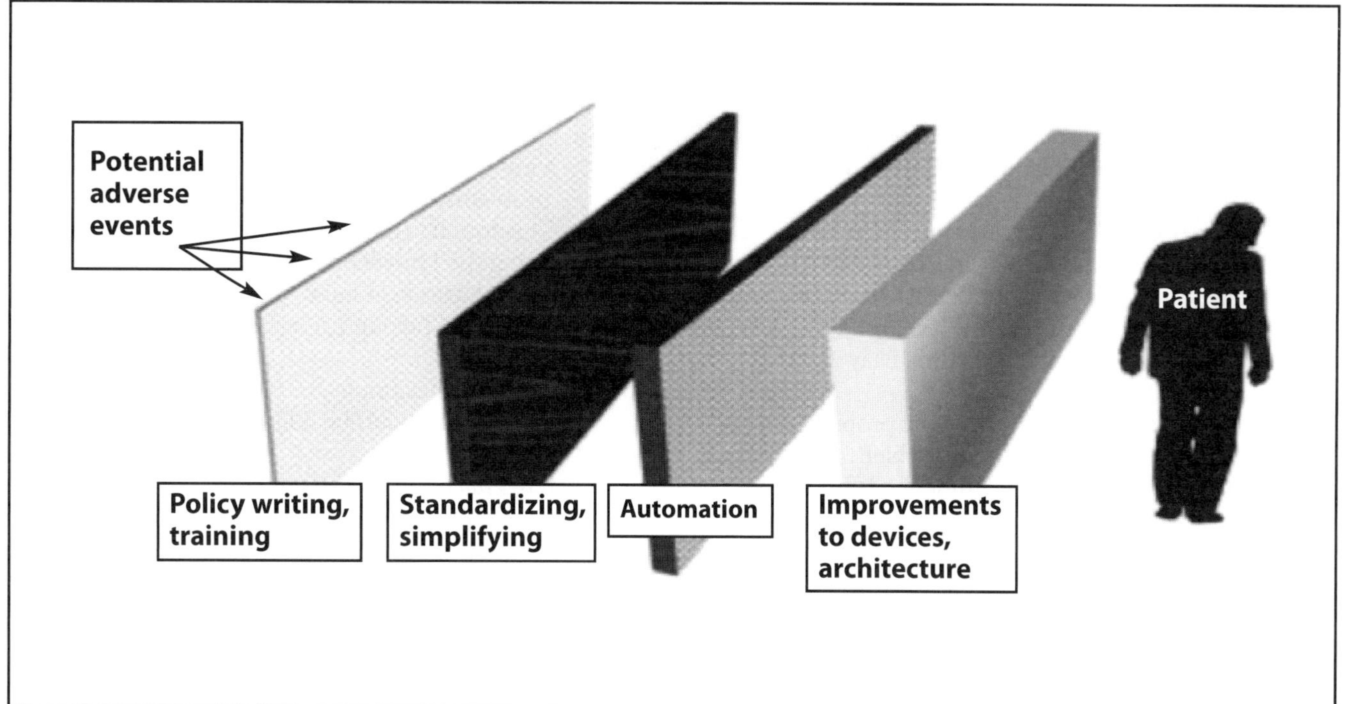

Figure 1.7. Protective effectiveness comparison. Notice that training and writing policies are the least effective barriers protecting patients from potential harm and that the level of protection increases with standardization and automation. This illustration also supports the goal to not blame staff when systems fail. *Used with permission from the Veteran's Administration.*

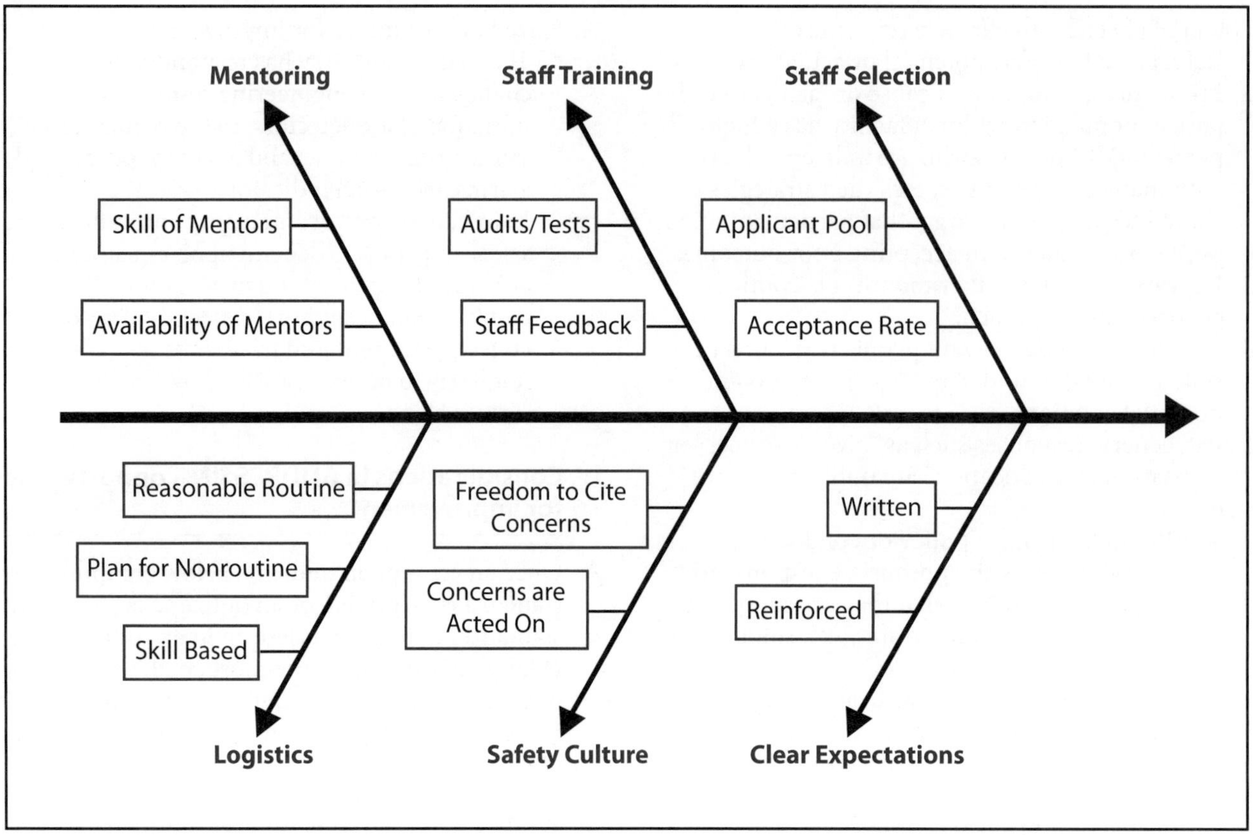

Figure 1.8. The Ishikawa or "fishbone" cause and effect diagram to analyze prescription errors.

1. These protective layers include staff selection, staff training, staffing model, staff auditing and support, plant and equipment protections, patient engagement, team safety net, and management oversight.
2. Each protective layer has vulnerabilities that can provide a route for error or failure to reach or nearly reach the level of patient harm.
3. Rosemarie Miller, a member of CMS's ESRD Survey Training and Support Team, calls this "route cause analysis," noting that reinforcement of system safeguards may be required on several levels (personal communication, May 2, 2012).

C. Conducting effective analysis of the problem often requires the use of a number of problem identification techniques to guide the team in collection of all information necessary to formulate a response strategy and appropriate interventions. Basic tools include:
   1. The Ishikawa (fishbone) diagram, which has the advantage of promoting full team participation (Institute for Healthcare Improvement, 2014a).
      a. Link to an example: http://www.ihi.org/knowledge/Pages/Tools/CauseandEffectDiagram.aspx
      b. Figure 1.8 represents a sample fishbone used to analyze prescription errors.
   2. The Five Whys, made popular by Toyota's Performance Improvement (PI) program, which asks why the problem occurred, then why the first response to that question occurred, and so on – five times of asking "why."
      a. Provides a quick drill down through layers of vulnerability to a deeper problem or set of problems.
      b. This tool has the advantages of simplicity and using the knowledge of front-line people to bring hazards to light.
      c. It can also help in prioritization of solutions (Ries, 2012).
      d. Link to an example: http://www.youtube.com/watch?v=D9Mae3WWVas
   3. Pareto charting (and histograms and frequency plots of all types) lend themselves well to addressing low performance on clinical outcome measures by plotting the frequency of specific problems (ASQ, n.d.).
      a. Link to an example: http://asq.org/learn-about-quality/cause-analysis-tools/overview/pareto.html
      b. The Pareto diagram explicitly provides information about the percentage of a problem cluster caused by ranked order factors, but a simple frequency diagram may provide all the

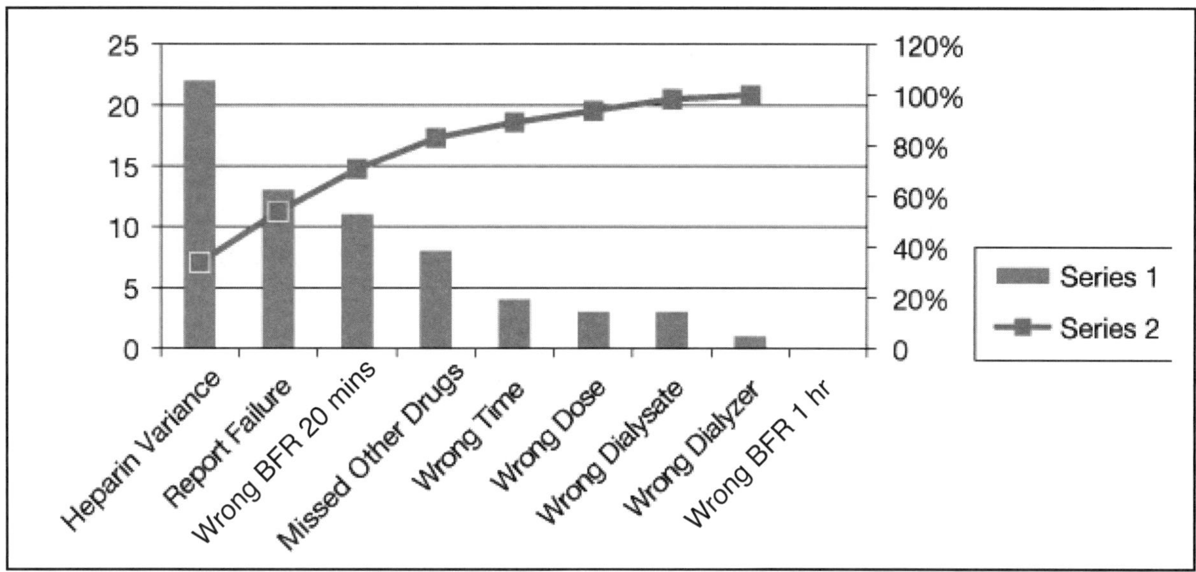

Figure 1.9. The Pareto diagram.

visual information required for priority setting.

c. This tool has the advantage of focusing efforts on the particular problems that, if corrected, could achieve the greatest improvement in the overall outcome measure.

d. For example: to evaluate patients not reaching expected base weight:
   (1) Identify the number of patients whose treatments could not be programmed for desired loss because it would result in weight loss greater than 15 mL/kg/hr.
   (2) Identify patients whose treatments were incorrectly programmed.
   (3) Identify patients who exhibited clinical symptoms and whose treatments had to be reprogrammed, and so on.
   (4) The counts might guide prioritization of intervention.

e. See Figure 1.9 for an example of a Pareto diagram.

4. Flow diagrams. These can be used to map or track processes through their cycle to find where breakdowns occurred. These diagrams can be useful in groups that are familiar with their use, but must be clearly constructed or they present the risk of creating a layer of complexity that prevents some staff members with crucial knowledge from easily contributing that knowledge. Figure 1.10 is an example of a confusing flow diagram.
5. Advanced tools, like Process Failure Mode Effect, can be used when a major new process is being implemented. These advanced tools each help build a path between the goal and the current status that identifies and manages the effect of system vulnerabilities (Institute for Healthcare Improvement, 2014b).
   a. Link for process failure mode effect examples: http://www.ihi.org/knowledge/Pages/Tools/FailureModesandEffectsAnalysisTool.aspx
   b. Link for a gap analysis tool: http://www.ahrq.gov/professionals/systems/hospital/qitoolkit/d5-gapanalysis.pdf

D. Addressing QAPI issues that have been identified requires team member acceptance of accountability for individual roles in action plan. As an illustration:
   1. A social worker and a physician meet with shift supervisors regarding six patients who have "at-risk" Kidney Disease Quality of Life (KDQOL) scores.
   2. They will develop strategies and input support reminders into the electronic medical record within the week.
   3. The nurse manager will follow up on any obstacles to implementation in 2 weeks.
   4. The physician and social worker will discuss the progress with the targeted patients during weekly rounds. This continues for 2 months.
   5. The six patients retest in 2 months. The social worker will report the results to QAPI team at their next meeting.

E. Timelines (as in the example above).
   1. It is important to develop a timeline for implementation.
   2. It is equally important to develop a timeline for evaluating the success of the strategies or needed revisions (CMS, 2008b).

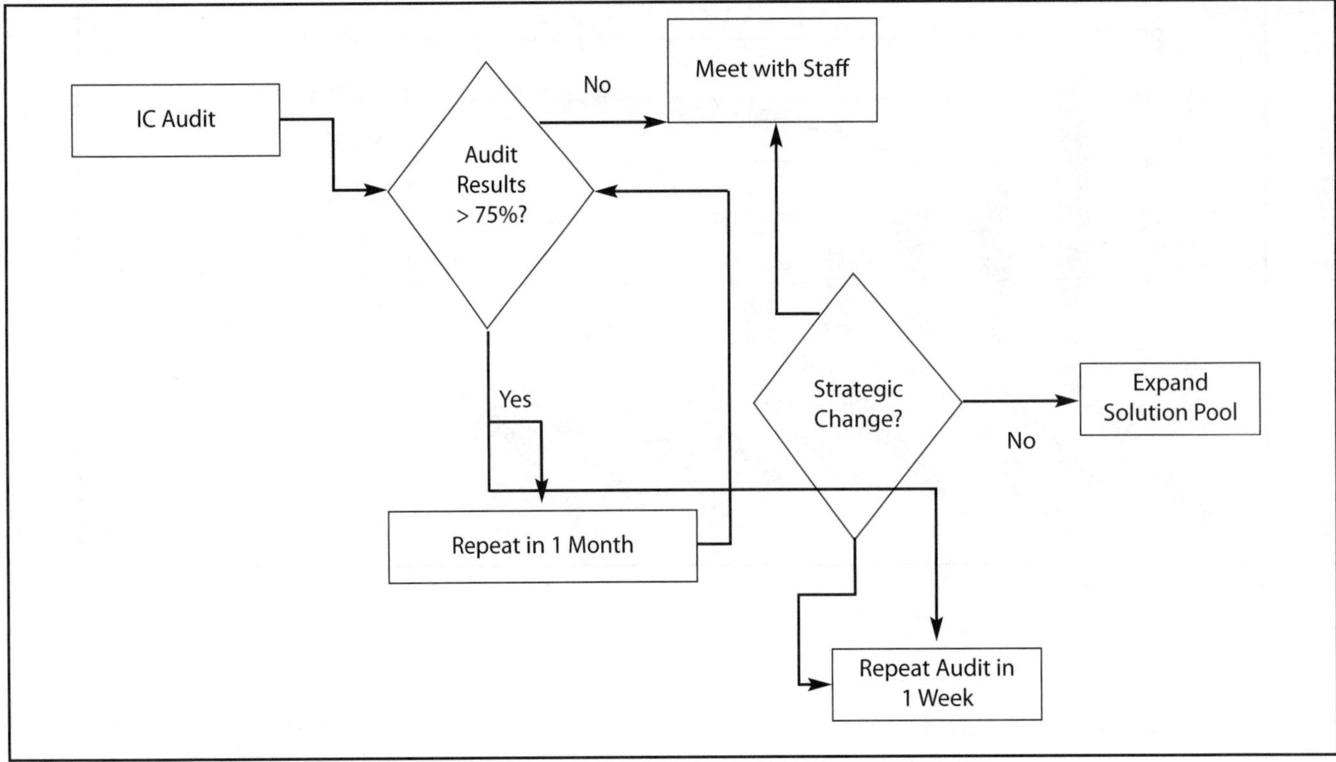

Figure 1.10. A confusing flow diagram.

F. Development of success metrics:
   1. How does one tell if action worked?
   2. How long will "success" be trended?
   3. How soon will the plan be revised if goal metrics are not achieved?

G. Scheduled evaluation of effectiveness of response strategy.

H. Establishing an ongoing, active, monitoring schedule (frequency of monitoring will be dependent on severity and extent of problem). As an illustration:
   1. A response to a "spike" in access infections and poor results on an audit of cannulation practices might read:
      a. The infection control (IC) nurse will audit practice weekly for 4 weeks by observing seven different staff members each week.
      b. The IC nurse will problem-solve technique breaks with staff on the day of audit.
      c. If > 90% procedural adherence, begin 3 months of monthly audits of seven different staff. Again, problem-solve technique breaks with staff day of audit.
      d. If > 90% procedural adherence, begin quarterly audits.
      e. If at any point < 90% adherence is observed on audit, obtain additional resources and establish new monitoring schedule as indicated.
   2. This level of plan specificity may be routine (and quick) for experienced QAPI teams or may require a designated subteam to meet and develop the plan and notify the full QAPI team.
   3. Without a specific implementation plan, the problem was mentioned, not addressed.

I. The ANNA publication, *Applying Continuous Quality Improvement in Clinical Practice,* 2nd edition (2009), offers numerous tools and strategies specific to all kidney replacement settings (Axley & Robbins, 2009).

SECTION E
Culture of Safety
Bonnie B. Greenspan

I. Development of the concept of a culture of safety.

A. Definition.
   1. Nursing and safety literature embrace the definition of organizational culture as the values, beliefs, and norms that are important in the organization.
   2. *Webster's Third New International Dictionary* (1993) includes customs and superstition in the definition.

3. In attempting to drive cultural change, a useful aspect of organizational culture was identified in Schein's original and now classic work: "Culture is what a group learns over time as that group solves its problems of survival in an external environment and its problems of internal integration" (Schein, 1990, p. 111).

B. Developing a culture of safety entails relinquishing or replacing some of that "survival" learning. The reverberations following the Chernobyl nuclear power plant accident were sufficient to drive the nuclear industry, as well as other High Reliability Organizations (HROs), to adopt a new culture of safety that included the core characteristics listed below (Collins, 2010).

C. The Institute of Nuclear Power Operations, requiring a clear definition to determine if the goal was being met, defined the HRO safety culture as: "Professional leadership attitudes that manage hazardous processes such that risk of harm to process workers, the public, and the environment is continually maintained acceptably low, thereby maintaining stakeholder trust" (Collins, 2010).

D. Telltale reports in health care.
   1. The landmark Institute of Medicine report, *To Err Is Human: Building a Safer Health System* (Kohn et al., 2000) revealed that between 44,000 and 98,000 Americans die annually as a result of medical errors.
      a. This report created comparable reverberations in health care.
      b. Attempts to create the most effective culture of safety specific to the healthcare environment began in earnest.
   2. A 2010 report by the Office of Inspector General for Health and Human Services increased that estimate to 180,000 preventable deaths per year (Levinson, 2010).
   3. In 2013, a study by the *Journal of Patient Safety* raised the estimate to between 210,000 and 440,000 per year (James, 2013).
      a. This study used the global trigger tool.
      b. The tool uses clues, like stop medication orders or problematic laboratory reports, to focus the attention of medical record reviewers on potential errors (James, 2013).

II. Core characteristics of safety culture in HROs (Taylor, 2010).

A. Safety is a clearly recognized value.

B. Leadership for safety is clear.

C. Accountability for safety is clear.

D. Safety is integrated into all activities.

E. Safety is learning driven.

III. Key elements of a healthcare culture of safety (Barnsteiner, 2011).

A. The establishment of safety as an organizational priority. Examples of reinforcement and openness include:
   1. Patient safety assessments with follow up.
   2. Safety rounds with follow-up.
      a. Institute of Healthcare Improvement (IHI) WalkRounds™. http://www.ihi.org/resources/Pages/Tools/PatientSafetyLeadershipWalkRounds.aspx
      b. Quality and Safety WalkRounds™. http://www.hse.ie/eng/about/Who/qualityandpatientsafety/Clinical_Governance/CG_docs/QPSwalkarounds240513.pdf
   3. "Parking lot" for safety concerns with follow-up.

B. Teamwork inclusivity is the key.

C. Patient involvement.

D. Openness and transparency.

E. Accountability.

IV. Safety culture is characterized by (Barnsteiner, 2011):

A. Shared core values and goals.

B. Nonpunitive responses to adverse events and errors.

C. Promotion of safety through education and training.

V. Patient involvement in the culture of safety in health care.

A. Patient involvement is evolving from not only the consumers' push, but also from the providers' pull.
   1. There is still far to go to achieve the Institute of Medicine's goal of patient-centered care.
   2. The care that is "respectful of and responsive to individual patient preferences, needs, and values, and ensure(s) that patient values guide all clinical decisions" (IOM, 2001).

B. The 2007 National Safety Goal of the Joint Commission mandated that healthcare organizations "encourage patients' active involvement in their own care as a patient safety strategy" (Metules & Bauer, 2006).
   1. Subsequent national safety goals incorporate patient education and participation in specific areas of care such as anticoagulation therapy, prevention of surgical site infection, and medication safety (The Joint Commission, 2014).

2. Specifically this goal requires the provider to:
   a. Define and communicate the means for patients and their families to report concerns about safety. The critical piece that is often missing is encouragement of reporting and evaluation of the success with this approach.
   b. Communicate with patients about all aspects of their care, treatment, or services.
      (1) When patients know what to expect, they are more aware of the potential risks as well as the choices they can make.
      (2) Patients can be an important source of information about potential adverse events and hazardous conditions.

C. The Agency for Healthcare Research and Quality (AHRQ) (2012) reports that the efforts to engage patients have focused on three areas:
   1. Enlisting patients in detecting adverse events. *Example*: participating in dialyzer identification and dialysis prescription verification.
   2. Empowering patients to ensure safe care. *Example*: encouraging patients to become familiar with infection control policies and to communicate potential breaches to caregiver.
   3. Emphasizing patient involvement as a means of improving a culture of safety. This entails routine inclusion of patient input at any of a number of levels:
      a. In identifying and addressing safety concerns about existing processes.
      b. In safety analysis for new processes.

D. Challenges have arisen in maximizing the effect of patient engagement on error reduction.
   1. Like many healthcare workers, patients have participated in the historic healthcare culture for varying lengths of time and vary in the extent and aspects of increased engagement they embrace.
   2. The continuum between inviting and mandating participation is even less controllable than with the caregivers, and neither has proven simple.
   3. Exploring and exploiting the potential in its safety primer, *The Role of the Patient in Safety*, AHRQ (2012) points out some controversial issues:
      a. Error reports in surveys from patients, given after discharge, have importantly pointed out a number of previously unreported errors. However, some argue that these reports center on service concerns more than clinical errors.
      b. Some patients have reported concerns about participation in ways that may appear (or actually become) confrontational, such as asking caregivers to wash their hands, although patient participation in this area has been reported to increase adherence.
      c. Expansion of patient participation could be increased through strong team development with patients located *inside* the team from the start and with the use of positive communication methods.

E. In 2010, Scobie and Persaud's proposed framework regarding how to engage patients in error prevention strategies listed several barriers and facilitators.
   1. Barriers include:
      a. Awareness: lack of awareness of risks, safety science, and terminology.
      b. Traditional patient/provider roles: reluctance to challenge, as discussed above.
      c. Self-efficacy: lack of role perception in this context.
      d. Healthcare setting and illness: comfort and health status can affect participation.
      e. Demographics: age, gender, and other factors may make engagement difficult or easier.
      f. Legality: effects on disclosure and liability.
   2. Facilitators include:
      a. When the providers and physicians modeled and instructed patients to ask questions of themselves and other providers, patients' willingness to do so improved.
      b. Increasing the patients' perception of risk by providing sufficient education about the potential harm of errors. This creates awareness and enough worry to motivate the patients to act on their own behalf.
      c. Willingness to participate, which is widely reported, should be met with appropriate education and support.

F. The Institute for Healthcare Improvement's Triple Aim of improving the patient experience of care and the health of populations while reducing per capita costs of health care has had success in incorporating engaged patients in all stages of program development. Success stories are chronicled at this site: http://www.ihi.org/offerings/initiatives/TripleAim/Pages/ImprovementStories.aspx

VI. Engaging healthcare workers.

A. It is imperative that healthcare workers (HCW) be engaged in bringing safety risks, and especially errors or near misses, to the attention of the team for analysis for improvement. The HCW must be able to do this without fear of potential repercussions.

B. "Just Culture" is the mechanism by which nonpunitive responses required for openness in error reporting and for system learning are reconciled with accountability.
   1. A *just culture* is one that "learns and improves by

examining its own weaknesses" (Frankel et al., 2006) and "is an atmosphere of trust in which people are encouraged, even rewarded, for providing essential safety information…but are clear about where the line must be drawn between acceptable and nonacceptable behavior" (Reason, 1997, p. 195).

2. A just culture attempts to address the appropriateness and system-wide effects of punitive response to errors. Shame and punishment of all errors results in failure to focus attention on system vulnerabilities and encourages concealment.
3. In January 2010, the American Nurses Association, in its Position Statement on Just Culture, asserted its support for the just culture concept and its application to nursing, moving away from health care's traditional culture, which "held individuals accountable for all errors or mishaps that befall patients under their care"(ANA, 2010b, p. 2).
4. While any movement away from the harsh and unrealistic error psychology that the traditional medical model frequently employed was a correction, more was needed to bring about the open reporting and examination of errors that a just culture was intended to support.
5. David Marx, an attorney, provided a basic structure for error classification and appropriate management response in 2001. He later refined the classification into a just culture algorithm to increase its effectiveness.
   a. For a just culture system to work, it requires:
      (1) Strict adherence by management to the conditions it put forth.
      (2) Sufficient clarity of those conditions to enable all staff to:
         (a) Understand the conditions.
         (b) Trust the system and all management to consistently implement it.
   b. Although Marx addressed a wide range of ethical and legal issues, to simplify: Marx aligned error types with management action.

C. Human error types. The current literature cites the following three error types that were identified by Marx (2001):
1. Inadvertent behavior (simple human error).
   Example: a hemodialysis HCW fails to turn on the blood pump to the prescribed flow rate at the initiation of the treatment resulting in inadequate dialysis.
2. At-risk behavior ("shortcut").
   Example: a hemodialysis HCW, in the interest of time, leaves the patient at a 200 blood flow rate (BFR) until the next patient treatment initiation is complete. The hemodialysis HCW then returns and increases the BFR on all assigned patients for that shift. This results in decreased adequacy of dialysis for each patient where implementation of the ordered BFR was delayed.
3. Reckless behavior (impaired, intentional disregard of unreasonable risk).
   Example: a hemodialysis HCW comes to work under the influence of alcohol (or angry and acting out at the person who made the assignment) and leaves the assigned patients at 200 BFRs and fails to monitor the patients' status for the duration of the treatment. This results in decreased dialysis adequacy for all and a drop in blood pressure for one of the patients.

D. Management considerations (ANA, 2010b).
1. Human error.
   a. Use normal error reduction techniques (e.g., simplification, improved training, re-engineering).
   b. Marx approach to individual: console.
2. At-risk behavior.
   a. Introspection and action on incentives and leadership messaging; manage value conflicts.
   b. Marx approach to individual: coach.
3. Reckless behavior.
   a. Remedial action or punishment; review vulnerabilities in supervision.
   b. Marx approach to individual: punish.

E. Distinct from an error, intentional or willful behavior requires the agency to analyze the reason for and appropriateness of the willful violation. This analysis could result in anything from revision of policy and procedure to reporting action to appropriate criminal authorities as indicated.

F. Decision tree for each of the three levels.
1. Although every error has more context than provided here, the basis for the response would not be primarily the effect on the patient(s).
2. Meadows, Baker, and Butler (2005) describe the use of a four-question incident decision tree consistent with the Marx algorithm to help determine how to categorize and respond to an error.
   a. The deliberate harm test.
      (1) Were the actions intended?
      (2) If yes, punitive action, as well as review for improved safety, is justified.
   b. The physical/mental health test.
      (1) Does there appear to be ill health or substance abuse?
      (2) If there appears to be substance abuse, personal accountability as defined by the individual system guidelines could justify punitive action.

c. The foresight test.
   (1) Did the individual break protocol?
   (2) Did the individual know the protocol?
   (3) Did the individual have access to the protocol and the supplies/equipment necessary to follow protocol?
   (4) Did the individual choose off-protocol action(s)? If individual took an unacceptable risk, as defined by the individual system guidelines, there may be justification for punitive action.
d. The substitution test.
   (1) Would a comparably educated and experienced individual be likely to behave the same way in similar circumstances?
   (2) If not, were there deficiencies in training or supervision?
   (3) If not, and the individual took an unacceptable risk as defined by the system guidelines, there may be justification for punitive action.

VII. One of the most compelling reasons for using error reports and near misses to identify and initiate action to address both individual competence and system vulnerabilities is that errors can be not simply sharp end or blunt end, but both (Gregory & Kaprielian, 2005).

A. Sharp end errors in health care are those that occur at the hand of the practitioner, such as:
   1. Contamination of clean site.
   2. Infiltration of an access.
   3. Misreading or miswriting an order.
   4. Neglecting to turn on heparin pump.

B. Blunt end errors occur more remotely from the point of the error, such as:
   1. Failure to make sufficient supplies accessible for clean procedures.
   2. Poor training or assignment, or lack of support for new employees in cannulation.
   3. Poor ordering mechanisms or failure to provide a "distraction-free zone" for noting orders.
   4. Unrealistic scheduling.
   5. No safety check "moment" expected at initiation of treatment.

C. For nurses to participate effectively in error reduction, they must develop and use skills to address contributing factors at both the sharp and the blunt ends.
   1. The Quality and Safety Education for Nurses (QSEN) Project used the Institute of Medicine competencies as the starting point for their faculty, an advisory board, and representatives from 11 nursing organizations to define quality and safety competencies and the knowledge, skills, and attitudes to be developed in nursing graduate programs (Cronenwett et al., 2009).
   2. A sample of one of the competencies, Safety, is reprinted in Table 1.1. More information can be found at http://qsen.org/competencies

VIII. Obstacles to creating a culture of safety.

A. Many healthcare settings have an existing culture of long standing.
   1. Transitioning to a safety culture in which every member has equal standing to address safety issues means that while some will have gained status, some will have lost it. And some of those who have gained status may find the corresponding accountability daunting.
   2. As Edgar Schein described in his work on organizational culture over 30 years ago, the current culture in healthcare facilities reflects the strategies developed over time to address threats that have not likely disappeared. As the historic culture drops away, new strategies will emerge to address them by design or default (Schein, 1990).
   3. The development of effective teamwork, on the "To Do" list of many leaders in safety, may facilitate selection of safer strategies, as good teams outside health care made fewer errors and were associated with lower stress levels (Firth-Cozins, 2001).

B. Prioritizing safety can at times compete with other priorities such as efficiency and elimination of waste.
   1. Morath (2011) compares High Reliability Organizations (HROs) to healthcare environments and questions, for example, how the participation of all nuclear plant workers in the revision of all processes (including evaluation of equipment and supplies) compares to the experience of most HCW in process change. She notes that in HROs there is "awareness and sensemaking" at every level.
   2. Morath (2011) invites others to consider the impact of failing to include HCW to a similar extent on the healthcare environment's ability to optimize individual benefit, system performance, and safety.

C. The constraints on blunt end of errors come despite the critical role Morath attributes to nurses in reducing sharp end errors, particularly when at-risk behaviors serve individual values in the short term (e.g., shortcuts can save time for the staff and often reduce direct expenses for the provider).
   1. As corner-cutting practices are accepted by the group, the safety boundary moves increasingly into the risk zone.

Table 1.1

Sample Competency from the Institute of Medicine's Competencies for Nursing Used by the Quality and Safety Education for Nurses (QSEN) Project

Safety		
Definition: Minimizes risk of harm to patients and providers through both system effectiveness and individual performance.		
Knowledge	**Skills**	**Attitudes**
Describe human factors and other basic safety design principles as well as commonly used unsafe practices (such as workarounds and dangerous abbreviations). Describe the benefits and limitations of selected safety-enhancing technologies (such as barcodes, computer provider order entry, and electronic prescribing). Evaluate effective strategies to reduce reliance on memory.	Participate as a team member to design, promote, and model effective use of technology and standardized practices that support safety and quality. Participate as a team member to design, promote, and model effective use of strategies to reduce risk of harm to self and others. Promote a practice culture conducive to highly reliable processes built on human factors research. Use appropriate strategies to reduce reliance on memory (such as forcing functions, checklists).	Value the contributions of standardization and reliability to safety. Appreciate the importance of being a safety mentor and role model. Appreciate the cognitive and physical limits of human performance
Delineate general categories of errors and hazards in care. Identify best practices for organizational responses to error. Describe factors that create a just culture and culture of safety. Describe best practices that promote patient and provider safety in the practice specialty.	Communicate observations or concerns related to hazards and errors to patients, families, and the healthcare team. Identify and correct system failures and hazards in care. Design and implement microsystem changes in response to identified hazards and errors. Engage in a systems focus rather than blaming individuals when errors or near misses occur. Report errors and support members of the healthcare team to be forthcoming about errors and near misses.	Value own roles in reporting and preventing errors. Value systems approaches to improving patient safety in lieu of blaming individuals. Value the use of organizational error reporting systems.

Source: Cronenwett, L., Sherwood, G., Pohl, J., Barnsteiner, J., Moore, S., Sullivan, D., Ward, D. & Warren, J. (2009). Quality and safety education for advanced nursing practice. *Nursing Outlook, 57*(6), 338-348. Accessed from http://qsen.org/competencies/graduate-ksa/ *Used with permission.*

2. To stand up for safety, the nurse must at some point push back against production and financial barriers (Morath & Turnbill, 2010).

IX. Resources in the pursuit of greater safety.

A. The End-Stage Renal Disease Network Collaborative and Five Diamond Program/Renal Physician's Association (RPA) Patient Safety Program – http://www.esrdnet5.org/Dialysis-Providers/5-Diamond-Program.aspx
   1. Designed for dialysis priorities.
   2. Provides 13 safety education modules with process assistance.
   3. Provides a model safety policy.
   4. Supports participation in the Centers for Disease Control (CDC) National Health Safety Network (NHSN).

B. The website for the Institute for Healthcare Improvement (http://www.ihi.org) includes "Changes For Improvement," free online classes on a wide array

of topics such as principles of safety, WalkRounds™, teamwork development, and an online menu of tips on the following recommendations:
1. Conduct patient safety leadership walk rounds.
2. Create a reporting system.
3. Designate a patient safety officer.
4. Reenact real adverse events from your facility.
5. Involve patients in these safety initiatives.
6. Appoint a safety champion.
7. Simulate possible adverse events.
8. Conduct safety briefings.
9. Create an adverse event response team.

C. The Agency for Healthcare Research and Quality (http://www.ahrq.gov). resources include:
1. Surveys on patient safety culture for use by providers.
2. Data, statistics, and tools.
3. Research findings and reports.
4. Fact sheets.

SECTION F
Role of Regulatory Agencies
Glenda M. Payne

I. The role of regulatory agencies.

A. State and federal regulations impact the practice of nephrology nurses. Nephrology is a highly regulated environment, with specific regulations for outpatient dialysis facilities and transplant programs.

B. Licensure.
1. At the time of publication, approximately 30 states had state-specific outpatient dialysis facility licensing rules and regulations.
2. In these states, outpatient facilities must have a state license to operate and cannot admit a patient until that license is obtained.
3. State licensure requirements may simply mirror the Medicare ESRD Conditions for Coverage (CfC) or may be more prescriptive and specific than the CfC.
4. Facilities are required to meet the more stringent requirement.

C. Medicare certification.
1. Transplant units and outpatient dialysis facilities must achieve and maintain Medicare certification to receive payment for the care they provide to Medicare beneficiaries.
2. To achieve and maintain certification, the transplant unit must meet the requirements outlined in the Conditions of Participation (CoP) for Hospitals and the Special Requirements for Transplant Centers: https://www.cms.gov/Medicare/Provider-Enrollment-and-Certification/Certificationand Complianc/downloads/Transplantfinal.pdf
3. The outpatient dialysis facility must meet the requirements outlined in the CfC for ESRD, which were completely revised in 2008: https://www.cms.gov/Regulations-and-Guidance/Legislation/CFCsAndCoPs/downloads/esrdfinalrule0415.pdf (CMS, 2008a).

D. Accreditation.
1. At the time of publication, there were four private agencies (listed below) that could bestow "deemed status" for hospital accreditation.
   a. "Deemed status" means that by successfully passing a survey conducted by one of these agencies, the hospital is "deemed" to meet the Medicare hospital CoP (Conditions of Participation).
   b. The hospital is then exempt from routine state or federal surveys.
2. By law, the "deemed status" applies to the general hospital requirements only, not to any ESRD program. The legislation which established the ESRD program specifically prohibits the application of "deemed status" to ESRD programs.
   a. In accredited hospitals, their "deemed status" does not apply to the kidney transplant program or any outpatient dialysis facility that might be a part of that hospital.
   b. The accredited hospital's transplant program and/or outpatient dialysis facility are subject to survey by the state agency for the applicable Medicare CoP for Hospitals and Special Requirements for Transplant Centers or the ESRD CfC.
3. Transplant programs and acute dialysis services are included in accreditation surveys and are expected to meet the requirements of the hospital's accreditation agency.
4. Accreditation agencies with "deemed status" for hospitals.
   a. The Joint Commission (TJC): http://www.jointcommission.org
   b. Health Care Facilities Accreditation Program (HFAP) of the American Osteopathic Association (AOA): http://www.hfap.org
   c. DNV GL Healthcare USA, Inc.: http://dnvglhealthcare.com/accreditations/hospital-accreditation
   d. Center for Improvement in Healthcare Quality (CIHQ): http://www.cihq.org

II. Conditions for Coverage for ESRD.

A. To be reimbursed for routine, repetitive, outpatient dialysis in a facility or at home, compliance with the Medicare ESRD Conditions for Coverage must be demonstrated.
   1. No payment is available for the treatment of Medicare beneficiaries until an initial survey for compliance with the ESRD CfC has been successfully completed.
   2. In 2013, CMS revised the routine ESRD survey process to a "Core" survey that reduces the time required for the survey while at the same time focusing on areas of highest risk for poor patient outcomes (CMS, 2013a).
      a. The focus of the CMS Core survey includes the following themes:
         (1) Data use. The survey process uses facility-specific and patient-specific data to both focus the survey and to evaluate process in areas where improvement is needed.
         (2) Infection control. The second highest cause of death in patients on dialysis is infection and the dialysis procedure offers many opportunities for cross contamination. A routine part of every survey is observation of infection control practices, with an expectation that each facility routinely monitors these practices as well.
         (3) QAPI. The Core survey includes an expectation that each facility actively monitors its own practices and takes action when improvement is needed or a potential for error or harm is identified.
      b. The following threads run throughout the ESRD Core survey:
         (1) Culture of safety.
            (a) Is there an open, transparent environment that encourages and supports reporting of errors and potential errors?
            (b) See the section in this chapter on Culture of Safety for more information on this topic.
         (2) Safety of dialysis delivery.
            (a) The technical aspects of the provision of dialysis (e.g., water treatment, dialysate preparation, machine operation and maintenance) present many potential risks to patient safety.
            (b) The Core survey uses a focused approach on critical requirements to ensure safe care is routinely delivered.
         (3) The patient's voice.
            (a) Patients are interviewed to determine if the facility care team actively engages the patient in his/her care and considers the patient's wishes and goals as paramount in designing the plan of care.
            (b) The facility is also expected to consider the patient's perspective in facility operations.

B. Prioritizing facilities for survey.
   1. CMS would prefer that each dialysis facility be surveyed at least every 3 years.
      a. However, most states do not have the personnel or financial resources to achieve that frequency.
      b. Therefore, CMS provides each state a rank-ordered list of their dialysis facilities using data from the Dialysis Facility Reports to include outcomes such as mortality, hospitalization rates, anemia management, and vascular access types.
   2. All facilities in the state are included in the list, with those facilities with the lowest outcomes listed first. States are required to choose a 10% sample of the facilities in their state, and must choose facilities in the first 20% of this list (i.e., facilities with the lowest outcomes).
   3. These surveys are considered the highest priority of any ESRD survey and thus likely to be conducted.

C. Using data to focus the survey.
   1. Once a facility is chosen for survey, the state surveyor is required to use that facility's patient outcomes to focus the survey.
   2. Surveyors review the facility's most recent Dialysis Facility Report (DFR), comparing the facility's outcomes with the average outcomes for each measure for the state, the Network, and the nation.
   3. Measures with lower outcomes are made a survey focus, unless current data shows improvement.
      a. Example one: If a facility's DFR outcomes show a higher percentage of patients who died or were hospitalized related to infection, the surveyor will consider infection as a focus. Infection control practices will be closely observed, the patient sample will include patients who have had infections, and QAPI will be reviewed for action plans to improve this outcome. If the facility has an effective action plan in place to reduce infections, any deficiencies cited would be tempered by the facility's efforts to address the problem.
      b. Example two: If a facility's DFR outcomes show a higher percentage of patients with hemoglobin levels less than 10 g/dL, the surveyor will plan to focus on anemia management. The focus will include patients with low hemoglobin levels in the sample and

QAPI activities in anemia management. When the surveyor arrives at the facility and reviews current data, if evidence of an effective plan to improve anemia management is presented, as well as laboratory reports showing a decrease in the number of patients with hemoglobin levels below 10 g/dL, the surveyor will remove "anemia management" from the list of data-driven survey focus areas.

D. How to prepare for an outpatient dialysis survey.
  1. Become familiar with the requirements. In addition to the federal regulations, determine if your state has ESRD licensing rules. If so, compare the state rules with the federal regulations. The more stringent requirement must be met.
    a. Example one: The federal regulations do not include specific staffing ratios, while several states mandate specific staff to patient ratios. If your state rules include a specific staffing ratio, you must meet that ratio or risk being cited for a deficient practice at both the federal and the state levels.
    b. Example two: Several states restrict what tasks patient care technicians (PCTs) may perform and may not allow PCTs to administer heparin or normal saline as part of the hemodialysis treatment.
  2. Know what is happening in the back room.
    a. Water treatment, dialysate preparation, and machine maintenance are areas that can present grave risks to patient safety.
    b. While the medical director is ultimately responsible for these and other areas of dialysis care, the nurse manger as well as designated members of the nursing staff must be competent in the monitoring of these systems.
  3. Recognize that plans of care are not about paper or complex electronic forms.
    a. Review of plans of care should demonstrate that the care team listens to the patient's wishes and goals and puts those first.
    b. Any member of the interdisciplinary team can update the plan of care to address progress or a change in the plan.
  4. Observe care.
    a. Recognize that the surveyor will expect to see that audits of care practices (e.g., initiation and termination of treatment and testing of water for total chlorine) are done for each staff member responsible for such tasks on at least an annual basis, and more frequently when problems in performance are identified.
      (1) The CMS Core survey includes guides for auditing practice. These are available in the ESRD Core Survey Field Manual: http://www.cms.gov/Medicare/Provider-Enrollment-and-Certification/GuidanceforLawsAndRegulations/Dialysis.html
      (2) Use of these tools provides a great way to stay "survey ready."
    b. Recognize that in-house, random audits initially conducted more frequently and then less frequently as practice improves, may be very effective in sustaining compliance to expected practice.
  5. QAPI.
    a. The Core survey process instructs surveyors to compare their findings with the facility's work in QAPI.
    b. If the facility has identified the same problem(s) and has an effective plan of improvement in place, citation of the problem under QAPI is likely unwarranted. (See the section on QAPI in this chapter for a more robust description of an effective QAPI program.)

III. Survey expectations for kidney transplant programs.

A. To be reimbursed for kidney transplants to Medicare beneficiaries, a transplant hospital must meet the CMS Conditions of Participation (CoP) for Hospitals and the Special Requirements for Transplant Centers.
  1. Transplant surveys are data driven.
    a. Transplant outcomes and complications are required to be reported and are reviewed quarterly by CMS staff.
    b. A drop in outcomes can result in a request for more information or an onsite survey by surveyors contracted for these surveys by CMS or the CMS Regional Office.
  2. Focused QAPI (fQAPI) surveys are abbreviated surveys directed at aspects of the transplant program's internal monitoring programs. An fQAPI survey may be done in response to data reports of negative outcomes or a specific complaint.

B. How to prepare for a survey of a kidney transplant unit.
  1. Become familiar with the requirements.
    a. Transplant units are required to be in compliance with the general hospital CoP as well as the Special Requirements for Transplant Centers.
    b. The survey of the transplant service focuses on the Special Requirements for Transplant. However, if noncompliance with the general CoP is identified, these deficient practices will be cited as well.
    c. Work with the hospital compliance department to become familiar with any previous Medicare surveys.

d. Use these URLs to access the interpretive guidance:
   (1) For the hospital CoP: http://www.cms.gov/Regulations-and-Guidance/Guidance/Manuals/downloads/som107ap_a_hospitals.pdf
   (2) For the transplant requirements: http://www.cms.gov/Medicare/Provider-Enrollment-and-Certification/GuidanceforLawsAndRegulations/Downloads/SurveyCertLetterInterpretiveGuidance.pdf
2. Ensure all required team members are providing the minimum expected care. The transplant CoP requires that the multidisciplinary team caring for kidney transplant recipients and living donors include representatives from the following disciplines:
   a. Medicine (transplant surgeon or transplant physician).
   b. Nursing.
   c. Social services.
   d. Clinical transplant coordinator.
   e. Nutrition.
   f. Pharmacology.
   g. Living donor advocate or advocate team.
3. Pay attention to outcomes. To be acceptable, the observed patient and graft survival rates for adult and pediatric kidney programs must to be equal to or better than expected survival rates (CMS, 2008c).
4. Communication is critical, including with:
   a. Patients on the waiting list.
   b. Referral centers such as dialysis facilities.
5. QAPI.
   a. The transplant program's QAPI work must include key personnel and an outcome and a process improvement project for each phase of the program (i.e., pretransplant, transplant/donation, and posttransplant) that are transplant-specific.
   b. If the transplant QAPI work is separate from the general hospital QAPI, the efforts and results must be communicated to the hospital's QAPI program. (See the section on QAPI in this chapter; for more information about transplant, see Module 3, Chapter 1.)

IV. Survey expectations for acute dialysis.

A. Accreditation entity requirements.
   1. TJC, HFAP, DNV GL Healthcare USA, Inc., and CIHQ survey hospitals for compliance with their standards, which must meet or exceed Medicare requirements.
   2. While these surveys may include acute dialysis services, there is little to no specific guidance in the accreditation manuals provided by the four agencies that have "deemed status" for hospitals.
   3. In 2013, one large dialysis organization submitted their acute programs for review under The Joint Commission's Ambulatory Care accreditation program with some dialysis-specific expectations added (Kulczycki, 2014).
      a. This accreditation applies to the system and is based on survey of a 25% sample of the participating dialysis sites.
      b. This program does NOT review for compliance with TJC hospital standards or the Medicare CoP for hospitals.
      c. This program does not provide deemed status.
      d. Acute dialysis services provided internally (rather than by contract) are not eligible for this accreditation.

B. Medicare Conditions of Participation (CoP) for Hospitals.
   1. In July 2013, CMS revised the hospital CoP for Discharge Planning to include expectations for the coordination of care for patients on dialysis transitioning from hospital to outpatient dialysis care.
   2. While this is the only area of the CoPs that specifically mentions dialysis, the following Conditions and Standards apply to the acute dialysis program:
      a. CoP: Governing Body.
         Example: The governing body of the hospital is responsible for the acute HD services offered in a hospital. If deficient practices in the acute HD service threaten the health and safety of patients, the CoP of Governing Body could be found out of compliance.
      b. Standard under CoP: Patient Rights.
         Example: The patient has a right to a safe environment. This requirement can be applied broadly and cited for any issue that presents a risk to the safety of patients receiving dialysis.
      c. CoP: QAPI.
         Example: The acute HD service is expected to have a robust QAPI program that reports to the overall hospital program. This requirement applies whether the acute HD service is provided by contract or by hospital employees.
      d. CoP: Nursing Services.
         Example: This CoP could be found out of compliance if personnel in use in the acute HD service were not qualified by experience or training for tasks they were assigned.
      e. Standards under CoP: Medical Record Services.
         Example: Annual review of any standing orders or protocols is expected.
      f. Standards under CoP: Pharmaceutical Services.
         Example: Medications must be stored in a secure area, and medications past their expiration dates are promptly removed from potential use.

g. CoP: Physical Environment.
Example: Problems in machine maintenance or the provision of safe water for dialysis could be cited here.
h. CoP: Infection Control.
Example: Ineffective infection control (i.e., poor hand hygiene, failure to immediately clean blood spills) and lack of tracking of elevated water or dialysate cultures or endotoxin testing could be cited here.
i. CoP: Discharge Planning.
Example: Lack of effective and timely discharge planning to include communication with the outpatient dialysis facility could be cited here.
j. Outpatient Services.
Example: This CoP would apply if the hospital offers outpatient dialysis to acute kidney injury patients. This CoP could be cited if such services are offered without policies and procedures to specify how these services are expected to be delivered, or if the outpatient dialysis service did not participate in QAPI.

C. How to prepare for a survey of an acute unit.
1. Become familiar with the requirements.
   a. Work with the hospital's accreditation coordinator to identify any areas identified as needing improvement in previous surveys and ensure these areas have been successfully addressed.
   b. Since each accreditation organization must ensure that the minimum standards outlined in the Medicare CoP for hospitals are met to retain the accrediting body's "deemed status," it is important to become familiar with the Medicare Conditions and Standards that apply to acute dialysis.
2. Become proficient with your water treatment system(s) and establish procedures that safely maintain them.
   a. If the hospital's general physical plant, engineering, or maintenance department is responsible for the water treatment systems, develop education materials and presentations to build competence in those staff members.
   b. Ensure tracking systems are in place to immediately identify any deviation from expected performance or outcomes.
3. Coordination of care.
   a. Provision of seamless transitions of patients from the inpatient dialysis unit to the nursing unit and to the outpatient dialysis facility is expected.
   b. Transfer of information is required from one point of care to the next, with receipt of this information expected prior to or at the time of arrival of the patient.
   c. This requirement is spelled out under the hospital CoP Discharge Planning, at tag A0837 in the Interpretive Guidelines.
   d. Cultivating relationships with referring outpatient dialysis facilities enables success in these efforts.
4. Observe care.
   a. Prevention of healthcare-associated infections must be a high priority.
   b. Nosocomial infections present a high risk for increased patient morbidity and mortality as well as potential financial loss for the hospital.
   c. Hand hygiene and strict practices for infection control are key to prevention of infection.
   d. The CDC developed audit tools and checklists to standardize and guide audits of practice. These are available at http://www.cdc.gov/dialysis/prevention-tools
5. QAPI.
   a. The acute hemodialysis program must participate in the hospital's QAPI program whether that service is provided by employees or by contract.
   b. The hospital employee assigned responsibility for supervision of the acute hemodialysis service must ensure a robust QAPI program is in place. (See the section on QAPI in this chapter for more information.)

References

Agency for Healthcare Research and Quality (AHRQ). (2008). *TeamSTEPPS. Implementation guide.* Retrieved from http://www.ahrq.gov/professionals/education/curriculum-tools/teamstepps/instructor/essentials/implguide.html

Agency for Healthcare Research and Quality (AHRQ). (2012). *Patient safety primers: Patient safety.* Retrieved from http://psnet.ahrq.gov/primer.aspx?primerID=17

Agency for Healthcare Research and Quality (AHRQ). (2013). *Multifaceted program increases reporting of potential errors, leads to action plans to increase safety.* AHRQ Health Care Innovations Exchange. Retrieved from http://partnershipforpatients.cms.gov/p4p_resources/tsp-culturechange/toolculturechange.html

Alexander, S. (1962, November 9). They decide who lives, who dies: Medical miracle and a moral burden of a small committee. *Life Magazine,* 102-125.

American Kidney Fund. (2014). *Weighing the outcomes: Ethical issues in kidney disease.* [Synched audio/slides] Retrieved from http: //www.prolibraries.com/anna/?select=session&sessionID=644

American Nephrology Nurses' Association (ANNA). (n.d.) *End of life decision-making and the role of the nephrology nurse.* Education Modules 1–4. (PowerPoint presentations). Retrieved from www.annanurse.org/resources/cne-opportunities /education-modules

American Nephrology Nurses' Association (ANNA). (2013). *ANNA position statement: Certification in nephrology nursing.* Retrieved from http://www.annanurse.org/download/reference/health /position/certNeph.pdf

American Nurses Association (ANA). (2010a). *Nursing: Scope and standards of practice* (2nd ed). Silver Spring, MD: Nursesbooks.org

American Nurses Association (ANA). (2010b). *Position statement: Just culture.* Congress on Nursing Practice and Economics. Retrieved from http://nursingworld.org/psjustculture

American Nurses Association (ANA). (2014). *Briefing paper on safe patient handling and mobility.* Retrieved from http://www.rnaction.org/site/DocServer/SPHM_w_Finance.pdf?docID=2001

American Society for Quality (ASQ) Knowledge Center (n.d.). *Cause analysis tools: Pareto diagram.* Retrieved from http://asq.org/learn-about-quality/cause-analysis-tools/overview/pareto.html

Axley, B., & Robbins, K.C. (2009). *Applying continuous quality improvement in clinical practice* (2nd ed.). Pitman, NJ: American Nephrology Nurses' Association.

Barnsteiner, J. (2011). Teaching the culture of safety. *The Online Journal of Issues in Nursing, 16*(3). doi:10.3912/ojin.Vol16No03Man05

Bennett, W. (2004). Ethical conflicts for physicians treating ESRD patients. *Seminars in Dialysis, 17*(1), 1-3.

Blackwell, L. (2011). Employee engagement in dialysis care, part 1: Understanding the disconnect. *Renal Business Today, 6*(4), 22-25.

Bosker, B. (2011, October 27). Cisco tech chief outlines the advantages of being a woman in tech. *The Huffington Post.* http://www.huffingtonpost.com/2011/10/27/cisco-chief-tech-officer-woman-in-tech_n_1035880.html

Boushey, H., & Glynn, S. (2012). *There are significant business costs to replacing employees.* Center for American Progress. Retrieved from http://www.americanprogress.org/issues/labor/report/2012/11/16/44464/there-are-significant-business-costs-to-replacing-employees/

Bozeman, B., & Fenney, M. (2007). Toward a useful theory of mentoring: A conceptional analysis and critique. *Administration and Society, 39*(6), 719-739. doi:10.1177100953997073041119

Campbell, G., Sanoff, S., & Rosner, M. (2010). Care of the undocumented immigrant in the United States with ESRD. *American Journal of Kidney Disease, 55*(1) 181-191.

Centers for Medicare & Medicaid Services (CMS). (2008a). *Conditions for coverage for end-stage renal disease facilities.* Final Rule, 73 Fed. Reg. 20481 (April 15, 2008) (42 CFR Parts 405, 410, 413 et al.).

Centers for Medicare & Medicaid Services (CMS). (2008b). *ESRD interpretive guidance* (Version 1.1). Retrieved from https://www.cms.gov/Medicare/Provider-Enrollment-and-Certification/SurveyCertificationGenInfo/downloads/SCletter09-01.pdf

Centers for Medicare & Medicaid Services (CMS). (2008c). *Organ transplant interpretive guidelines.* Retrieved from http://www.cms.gov/Medicare/Provider-Enrollment-and-Certification/GuidanceforLawsAndRegulations/Downloads/SurveyCertLetterInterpretiveGuidance.pdf

Centers for Medicare & Medicaid Services (CMS). (2013a). *Core survey field manual* (Version 1.6). Retrieved from http://www.cms.gov/Medicare/Provider-Enrollment-and-Certification/GuidanceforLawsAndRegulations/Dialysis.html

Centers for Medicare & Medicaid Services (CMS). (2013b). 42 CFR Parts 413 and 414. Medicare Program; *End-stage renal disease prospective payment system, quality incentive program, and durable medical equipment, prosthetics, orthotics, and supplies.* Final Rule. Retrieved from http://www.gpo.gov/fdsys/pkg/FR-2013-12-02/pdf/2013-28451.pdf

Centers for Medicare & Medicaid Services (CMS). (2014). *ESRD quality incentive program.* Retrieved from http://www.cms.gov/Medicare/Quality-Initiatives-Patient-Assessment-Instruments/ESRDQIP/

Centers for Medicare & Medicaid Services (CMS). (n.d.). *ESRD network organizations manual, chapter 9 – Grievances and patient-appropriate access to care and PCU enhancements.* Draft planned for 2015 publication.

Cherie, A., & Gebrekidan, A. (2005). *Lecture notes for nursing students: Nursing leadership and management.* Addis Ababa University. Retrieved from http://www.cartercenter.org

Cleaver, T. (2013, April 25). *The high (and hidden) costs of staff turnover in healthcare.* Retrieved from http://blog.shifthound.com/the-high-and-hidden-costs-of-staff-turnover-in-healthcare

Collins, D. (2010, January). *INPO HRO safety culture definition – An integrated approach.* Retrieved from http://www.nrc.gov/about-nrc/regulatory/enforcement/hro-sc-collins.pdf

Communication. (n.d.). In *Merriam-Webster's online dictionary* (11th ed.). Retrieved from http://www.merriam-webster.com/dictionary/communication

Covey, S. (2005a). *The 7 habits of highly effective people.* New York: Franklin Covey Co.

Covey, S. (2005b). *The 8th habit: From effectiveness to greatness.* New York: Free Press – Simon and Schuster.

Cronenwett, L., Sherwood, G., Pohl, J., Barnsteiner, J., Moore, S., Sullivan, D., … Warren, J. (2009). Quality and safety education for advanced nursing practice. *Nursing Outlook, 57*(6), 338-348.

Currier, H. (1994). Ethical issues in the neonatal patient with end stage renal disease. *Journal of Perinatal and Neonatal Nursing, 8*(1), 74-78.

Danis, M., & Hurst, S. (2009). Developing the capacity of ethics consultants to promote just resource allocation. *American Journal of Bioethics, 9,* 37-39.

Doyal, L., & Henning, P. (1994). Stopping treatment for end-stage renal failure: The rights of children and adolescents. *Pediatric Nephrology, 6,* 768-771.

ESRD Network Coordinating Center (NCC). (n.d.). *Homepage: About us, networks, patients, providers, resources, tools.* Retrieved from http://esrdncc.org

Fassett, R.G., Robertson, I.K., Mace, R., Youl, L., Challenor, S., & Bull, R. (2011). Palliative care in end-stage kidney disease. *Nephrology, 16*(1), 4-12. doi: 10.1111/j.1440-1797.2010.01409.x

Firth-Cozens, J. (2001). Cultures for improving patient safety through learning: The role of teamwork. *Quality in Health Care, 10*(Suppl. 2), ii26–ii31.

Fox, R.C., & Swazey, J. (1974). *The courage to fail: A social view of*
Chicago

t culture,
chieve
-1709.

ognized:
dialysis
39-253.
se a
from
/Pages/
or.aspx
of practice
ociation.
Duke

nets.html
g trapped
mmas in
hemodialysis care that evoke a troubled conscience. *BMC Medical Ethics, 12*(8). doi:10.1186/1472-6939-12-8

Hanson, D. (2014, January/February). Healthy work environments: Essential for innovation, transformation. *The American Nurse.* Retrieved from http://www.theamericannurse.org/index.php/2014/03/03/healthy-work-environments-essential-for-innovation-transformation/

Harari, O. (2002). *People over plans. The leadership secrets of Colin Powell.* New York: McGraw Hill.

Hijazi, F., & Holley, J. (2003). Cardiopulmonary resuscitation and dialysis: Outcome and patients' views. *Seminars in Dialysis, 16*(1), 51-53.

Husted, J., & Husted, G. (2008). *Ethical decision making in nursing and health care: A symphonological approach* (4th ed.). New York: Springer.

Institute for Healthcare Improvement. (2014a). *Cause and effect diagram.* Retrieved from http://www.ihi.org/knowledge/Pages/Tools/CauseandEffect Diagram.aspx

Institute for Healthcare Improvement. (2014b). *Failure modes and effects analysis* (FMEA) tool. Retrieved from http://www.ihi.org/knowledge/Pages/Tools/FailureModesand EffectsAnalysisTool.aspx

Institute of Medicine (IOM). (2001). *Crossing the quality chasm: A new health system for the 21st century.* Washington, DC: National Academy Press.

Institute of Medicine (IOM). (2010). *The future of nursing: Leading change, advancing health.* Retrieved from http://www.iom .edu/Reports/2010/The-future-of-nursing-leading-change-advancing-health.aspx

James, J.T. (2013). A new evidence-based estimate of patient harms associated with hospital care. *Journal of Patient Safety, 9*(3), 122-128.

Joffe, A. (2007). The ethics of donation and transplantation: Are definitions of death being distorted for organ transplantation? *Philosophy, Ethics, and Humanities in Medicine, 2*(28). doi:10.1186/1747-5341-2-28

Jonsen, A. (1998). *A short history of medical ethics.* New York: Oxford University Press.

Jonsen, A., Siegler, M., & Winslade, W (2006). *Clinical ethics: A practical approach to ethical decisions in clinical medicine* (6th ed.). New York: McGraw Hill Medical.

Kohn, L., Corrigan, J., & Donaldson, M., (Eds.). Committee on Quality of Health Care in America Institute of Medicine. (2000). *To err is human: Building a safer health care system.* Washington, D.C.: National Academy Press.

Kulczycki, M. (2014, October 13). *Standardization in acute hemodialysis programs: Joint Commission requirements.* Presented at the fall meeting of the American Nephrology Nurses' Association, Savannah, GA.

Lachman, V. (2006). *Applied ethics in nursing.* New York: Springer Publishing Co.

Lantos, J., & Warady, B. (2012). Should a nonadherent adolescent receive a second kidney? *Journal of the American Medical Association, 14*(3), 190-193.

Levinson, D. (2010). *Adverse events in hospitals: National incidence among hospital beneficiaries.* (OEI-06-09-00090). Report from the Office of Inspector General, DHHS. Washington, DC: U.S. Government Printing Office. Retrieved from http://oig.hhs.gov/oei/reports/oei-06-09-00090.pdf

Levinson, D. (2012). *Hospital incident reporting systems do not capture most patient harm.* (OEI-06-09-00091). Report from the Office of Inspector General, DHHS. Washington, DC: U.S. Government Printing Office. Retrieved from https://oig.hhs.gov/oei/reports/oei-06-09-00091.pdf

Longo, J., & Hain, D. (2014). Bullying: A hidden threat to patient safety. *Nephrology Nursing Journal,* 41(2), 193-199.

Lorenz, S., Bardon, O., & Vila Paz, M. (2008). Abstract: Patients in pre-dialysis decision taking and free choice of treatment (in English). *Nefrologia, 28*(Suppl. 3), 119-122.

Marx, D. (2001). *Patient safety and the "just culture": A primer for health care executives.* New York: Columbia University

Maxfield, D., Grenny, J., McMillan, R., Patterson, K., & Switzler, A. (2005). *Silence kills: The seven crucial conversations in healthcare.* VitalSmarts, AORN, & AACN. Retrieved from http://www.silenttreatmentstudy.com

Mazaris, E., Warrens, A., & Papalois, V. (2009). Ethical issues in live donor kidney transplant: Views of medical and nursing staff. *Experimental and Clinical Transplantation, 7*(1), 1-7.

McCormick, T. (1993). Ethical issues in caring for the patient with renal failure. *Nephrology Nursing Journal, 20*(5), 549-555.

Meadows, S., Baker, K., & Butler, J. (2005). The incident decision tree: Guidelines for action following patient safety incidents. In K. Henricksen, J. Battles, E. Marks, D.I. Lewin, & K. Henriksen (Eds.), *Advances in patient safety: From research to implementation* (Volume 4: Programs, tools, and products). Rockville, MD: Agency for Healthcare Research and Quality. Retrieved from http://www.ncbi.nlm.nih.gov/books/NBK20586

Medicare Improvements for Patients and Providers Act (MIPPA) of 2008. Pub. L. No. 110-275. Retrieved from http://www.gpo.gov/fdsys/pkg/PLAW-110publ275/pdf/PLAW-110publ275.pdf

Metules, T.J., & Bauer, J. (2006). JCAHO's patient safety goals, part 1: A practical guide. *Modern Medicine.* Retrieved from http://www.modernmedicine.com/modern-medicine/news/jcahos-patient-safety-goals-part-1-practical-guide

Mick J., Wood G., & Massey, R. (2007). The good catch pilot program: Increasing potential error reporting. *Journal of Nursing Administration, 37*(11), 499-503.

Miller, K. (1999). Ending renal dialysis: Ethical issues in refusing life-sustaining treatment. Life And Learning. IX: Proceedings of the Ninth University Faculty For Life Conference. Washington, DC.

Moore, L., Leahy, C., Sublett, C., & Lanig, H. (2013). Understanding nurse-to-nurse relationships and their impact on work environments. *MedSurg Nursing,* 22(3), 172-179.

Morath, J., & Turnbill, J. (2010). *To do no harm: Ensuring patient safety in health care organizations.* San Francisco: Jossey-Bass.

Morath, J. (2011). Nurses create a culture of patient safety: It takes more than projects. *The Online Journal of Issues in Nursing, 16*(3). doi:10.3912/OJIN.Vol16No03Man02

Moss, A. (2011). Time to talk about end-of-life care. *Nephrology Times, 4*(10), 3-4.

National Labor Relations Act. (1935). Retrieved from http://www.nlrb.gov/resources/national-labor-relations-act

Northouse, P. (2004). Team leadership. In S. Hill (Ed.). *Leadership: Theory and practice* (pp. 203-225). London: Sage.

O'Keefe, C. (2014). The authority for certain clinical tasks performed by unlicensed patient care technicians and LPNs/LVNs in the hemodialysis setting: A review. *Nephrology Nursing Journal, 41*(3), 247-255.

Professionalism (n.d.) In *Merriam-Webster's online dictionary* (11th ed.). Retrieved from http://www.merriam-webster.com/dictionary/professionalism

Reason, J. (1997). *Managing the risks of organizational accidents.* Aldershot, UK: Ashgate.

Renal Physicians Association (RPA). (2011). Shared decision making in the appropriate initiation of and withdrawal from dialysis (2nd ed.). Rockville, MD: Author.

Ries, E. (2012). To get to the root of a hard problem, just ask "why" five times. Retrieved from http://www.fastcodesign.com/1669738/to-get-to-the-root-of-a-hard- problem-just-ask-why-five-times

Rinehart, A. (2013). Beyond the futility argument: The fair process approach and time-limited trials for managing dialysis conflict. *Clinical Journal of the American Society of Nephrology, 8*(11), 2000-2006.

Ripley, E.B.D. (2009). Where does the nephrologist stand with a noncompliant, abusive dialysis patient? *International Journal of Nephrology, 5*(1).

Ritter, D. (2011). The relationship between healthy work environments and retention of nurses in a hospital setting. *Journal of Nursing Management, 19*, 27-32.

Rivin, A.U. (1997). Futile care policy: Lessons learned from three years' experience in a community hospital. *Western Journal of Medicine, 6*, 389-393.

Russ, A., Shim, J., & Kaufman, S. (2005). Is there life on dialysis? *Medical Anthropology, 24*(4), 297-324.

Russ, A., Shim, J., & Kaufman, S. (2007). The value of "life at any cost": Talk about stopping dialysis. *Social Sciences in Medicine, 64*(11), 2236-2247.

Sandberg, S. (2013). *Lean in: Women, work, and the will to lead.* New York: Alfred K. Knopf.

Schein, E. (1990). Organizational culture. *American Psychologist, 45*(2), 109-119. doi:10.1037/0003-066x.45.2.109

Scobie, A.C., & Persaud, D.D. (2010). Patient engagement in patient safety: Barriers and facilitators. *Patient Safety and Quality Healthcare.* Retrieved from http://www.psqh.com/marchapril-2010/454-patient-engagement-in-patient-safety-barriers-and-facilitator

Simmons, R.G. (1977). *Gift of life: The social and psychological impact of organ transplantation.* New York: John Wiley and Sons

Spital, A., & Taylor, J.S. (2007). Living organ donation: Always ethically complex. *Clinical Journal of the American Society of Nephrology, 2*(2), 203-204.

Studer, Q. (2003). *Hardwiring excellence.* Gulf Breeze, FL: Fire Starter Publishing.

Studer Group: Nursing and Physician Leaders from Across the Country (2010). *The nurse leader handbook: The art and science of nurse leadership.* Gulf Breeze, FL: Fire Starter Publishing.

Studer Group (n.d.). *Selecting talent behavioral interview guide, behavioral based interview questions, selecting and retaining talent: Tools for the bottom line.* Retrieved from https://www.studergroup.com/resources/learning-lab/results

Styles, M. (1982). *On nursing: Toward a new endowment.* St. Louis: Mosby.

Sullivan, J.D. (2010). End stage renal disease economics and the balance of treatment modalities. *Journal of Service Science and Management, 3*(1), 45-50.

Sutton, G., Liao, J., Jimmieson, N., & Restubog, S. (2011). Measuring multidisciplinary team effectiveness in a ward-based healthcare setting: Development of the team functioning tool. *Journal for Healthcare Quality, 33*(3), 10-25.

Tamura, M., Goldstein, M., & Perez-Stable, E. (2010). Preference for dialysis withdrawal and engagement in advance care planning within a diverse sample of dialysis patients. *Nephrology, Dialysis, and Transplantation, 25*(1), 237-242.

Taylor, J. (2010). *Safety culture: Assessing and changing the behavior of organizations.* Surrey, England: Gower Publishing Limited.

Templar, R. (2005). *The rules of management: A definitive code for managerial success.* New Jersey: Pearson Prentice Hall.

The Joint Commission. (2008). *Sentinel event alert: Behaviors that undermine a culture of safety.* Retrieved from http://www.jointcommission.org/assets/1/18/SEA_40.PDF

The Joint Commission. (2014). *National patient safety goals effective January 1, 2014.* Office-Based Surgery Accreditation Program. Retrieved from http://www.jointcommission.org/assets/1/6/OBS_NPSG_Chapter_2014.pdf

Tye, J. (2014). *The Florence prescription: From accountability to ownership* (2nd ed.). Solon, IA: Values Coach, Inc.

Ulrich, B. (2012). *Mastering precepting: A nurse's handbook for success.* Indianapolis: Sigma Theta Tau International.

U.S. Equal Opportunity Commission. (2014). *Enforcement guidance: Reasonable accommodation and undue hardship under American Disabilities Act.* Retrieved from http://www.eeoc.gov/policy/docs/accommodation.html

Veteran's Administration. (n.d.). *VA National Center for Patient Safety.* Retrieved from http://www.patientsafety.va.gov

Webster's third new international dictionary of the English language, abridged. (1993). Springfield, MA: Merriam-Webster.

Weinfield, R., & Donohue, E. (1989). *Communicating like a manager.* Baltimore: Williams and Wilkins.

White, D.B., Katz, M.H., Luce, J.M., & Lo, B. (2009). Who should receive life support during a public health emergency? Using ethical principles to improve allocation secisions. *Annals of Internal Medicine, 150*(2), 132-138.

Wolstenholme, G.E.W., & O'Connor, M. (1966). Problems of ethics in relation to haemo-dialysis and transplantation. In G.E. Schreiner (Ed.), *Ethics in medical progress: With special reference to transplantation* (pp. 126-133). Ciba Foundation Symposium. London: J & A Churchill Ltd. Retrieved from http://onlinelibrary.wiley.com/doi/10.1002/9780470719480.ch8/summary doi:10.1002/9780470719480.ch8

Note: There are 189,000 Google entries under the phrase *Bioethical Dilemmas in End Stage Renal Disease.* Numerous textbooks written by nurses, physicians, and bioethicists are available for review of bioethics principles and general aspects of decision making. Current books of case studies may not be useful because of the maturity of the ESRD specialty; they may no longer include dilemmas in ESRD care.

CHAPTER **2**

Research and Evidence-Based Practice in Nephrology Nursing

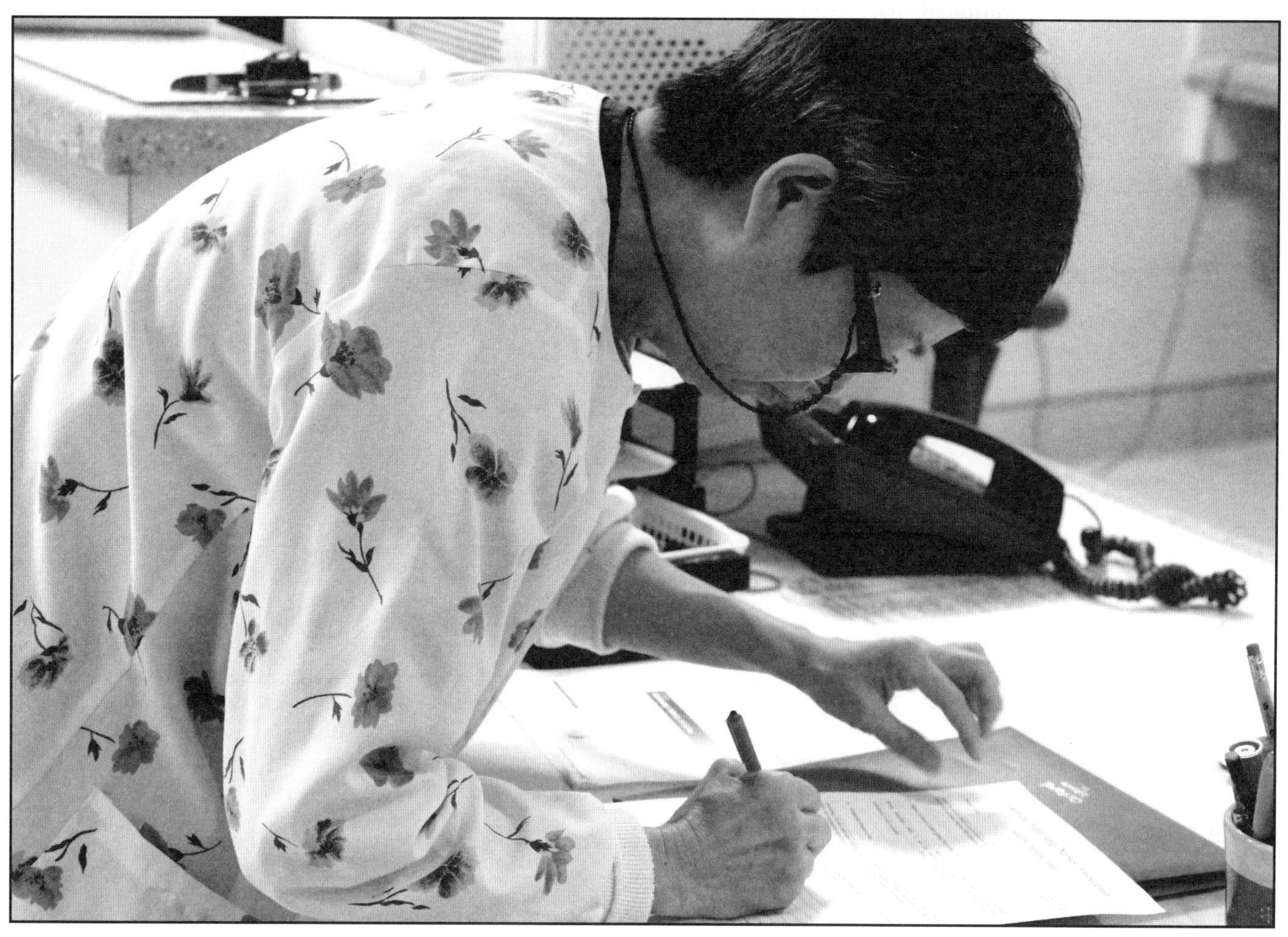

Chapter Editor
Tamara Kear, PhD, RN, CNS, CNN

Authors
Tamara Kear, PhD, RN, CNS, CNN
Caroline S. Counts, MSN, RN, CNN
Alicia M. Horkan, MSN, RN, CNN
M. Sue McManus, PhD, APRN, FNP-BC, CNN
Lisa Micklos, BSN, RN
Gail S. Wick, MHSA, BSN, RN, CNNe
Linda S. Wright, DrNP, RN, CNN, CCTC

CHAPTER 2
Research and Evidence-Based Practice in Nephrology Nursing

This offering for **1.5 contact hours** is provided by the American Nephrology Nurses' Association (ANNA).

American Nephrology Nurses' Association is accredited as a provider of continuing nursing education by the American Nurses Credentialing Center Commission on Accreditation.

ANNA is a provider approved by the California Board of Registered Nursing, provider number CEP 00910.

This CNE offering meets the continuing nursing education requirements for certification and recertification by the Nephrology Nursing Certification Commission (NNCC).

To be awarded contact hours for this activity, read this chapter in its entirety. Then complete the CNE evaluation found at **www.annanurse.org/corecne** and submit it; or print it, complete it, and mail it in. Contact hours are not awarded until the evaluation for the activity is complete.

Example of reference in APA format. Use author of the section being cited. This example is based on Section B – Standards for Care.

Micklos, L. (2015). Research and evidence-based practice in nephrology nursing: Standards for care. In C.S. Counts (Ed.), *Core curriculum for nephrology nursing: Module 1. Foundations for practice in nephrology nursing* (6th ed., pp. 63-86). Pitman, NJ: American Nephrology Nurses' Association.

Interpreted: Section author. (Date). Title of chapter: Title of section. In …

Cover photo by Counts/Morganello.

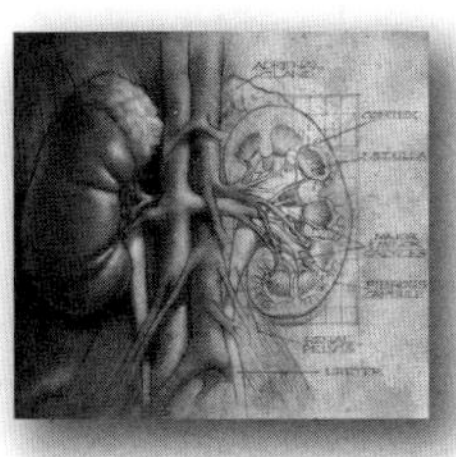

CHAPTER 2

Research and Evidence-Based Practice in Nephrology Nursing

Purpose

Using available evidence and research to make clinical decisions in nephrology nursing practice is essential for effective, efficient, and safe care delivery. This chapter begins with an introduction to research and evidence-based practice. There is a compare and contrast of evidence-based practice and research. The evolution and existing standards for nephrology nursing practice and interprofessional collaboration initiatives are discussed. The chapter concludes with KDOQI, KDIGO, DOPPS, USRD, CROWNWeb, and UNOS data, measures, and guidelines directing best practice.

Objectives

Upon completion of this chapter, the learner will be able to:

1. Describe the process used in establishing evidence-based practice.
2. Compare and contrast research utilization and evidence-based nursing practice.
3. Incorporate standards for care into clinical practice.
4. Discuss data, measures, and guidelines directing best practice in nephrology nursing.

SECTION A

Overview of Research and Evidence-Based Practice

Tamara Kear

I. What is evidence-based practice (EBP) and nursing research?

A. Historical background of EBP (Dearholt & Dang, 2012).
   1. Dates back to 1837 in Paris.
      a. EBP started by Dr. Pierre-Charles-Alexandre-Louis, a French physician.
      b. Dr. Pierre Louis analyzed the efficacy of bloodletting in the treatment of acute pneumonia.
   2. EBP movement: founded by British epidemiologist Archie Cochrane.
      a. In 1972, Dr. Cochrane published the book, *Effectiveness and Efficiency: Random Reflections on Health Science*. This book is thought to be the catalyst for the modern evidence-based practice movement.
      b. Encouraged public to pay only for empirically supported care.
      c. Criticized medical profession for not doing rigorous reviews of randomized controlled trials (RCTs) to assist others in making decisions about health care (e.g., policy makers and organizations).
      d. Established the foundation for initiation of the Cochrane Center, 1992 and Cochrane Collaboration, 1993.
         (1) Cochrane Library produced by worldwide virtual Cochrane Collaboration.
         (2) Prepares, maintains, and updates systematic reviews of interventions.
         (3) Ensures that reviews are accessible to the public.
   3. The Briggs Report published in the 1970s through the Department of Health and Social Security recommended that nursing become evidence-based.
      a. Professor Joanna Briggs reviewed the education and training of nurses and midwives in the United Kingdom.
      b. Professor Briggs reported that education was inadequate and basic nursing could only be learned in clinical settings.
      c. Proposed a two-tiered system leading to two levels of nurses, a large expansion in training and teaching, and a new statutory body.

   d. Six years of debate led to modified Briggs proposals and formed the basis of the Nurses, Midwives and Health Visitors Act of 1979.

B. Historical background of nursing research (Polit & Beck, 2012).
  1. Highlights prior to 1970.
     a. Nightingale's *Notes on Nursing.*
     b. Advent of nursing research journals such as *Advances in Nursing Science, Research in Nursing & Health, Western Journal of Nursing Research,* and *The Journal of Advanced Nursing.*
     c. Changes were occurring in nursing education, as more nurses were engaging in research and entering doctoral programs.
  2. The 1970s to 1990s.
     a. Research utilization projects focused on clinical practice issues and shifted from a prior focus on teaching, curriculum, and nurses' focus on researching themselves. Examples include quality of life, dietary behaviors, benefit of exercise regimens, self-care practices, and adequacy of the renal replacement therapy (RRT). *Note: RRT is now referred to as kidney replacement therapy (KRT).*
     b. Establishment of National Council for Nursing Research as an evolution from the National Institute for Nursing Research at the National Institutes of Health.
     c. Introduction of many additional nursing journals focusing on research.
     d. Cochrane Collaborative at Oxford formed to organize medical literature in a systematic manner for use by all health care practitioners.
     e. Formation of Agency for Healthcare Research & Quality (AHRQ) and National Quality Formum (NQF) to advance excellence, safety, standardized measurements, and quality in health care.
  3. Today and in the future.
     a. Focus on high quality evidence-based practice projects and interprofessional collaboration within companies, organizations, and places of higher learning.
     b. Increased focus on interprofessional research, too.
     c. American Association of Colleges of Nursing: Essentials Series for bachelor's, master's, and doctoral nursing programs: http://www.aacn.nche.edu/education-resources/essential-series

C. Similarities and differences between EBP and nursing research.
  1. Similarities.
     a. Each follows a systematic process and specific approach.
     b. Goal is to gain new knowledge related to an intervention or phenomenon.
  2. Differences.
     a. Research is more rigorous than EBP (Lee et al., 2013).
     b. Research tries to gain new knowledge.
     c. EBP takes knowledge produced by research and translates it into applicable practice and measures the effectiveness by evaluating outcomes (Lee et al., 2013).

D. Terminology commonly used in EBP resources and research articles.
  1. Bias is a distortion in study design, conduct of the study, or the outcomes that may cause a deviation from the truth (Polit & Beck, 2012).
  2. Clinical practice guidelines are evidence-based statements or statements supported by a systematic review of the evidence, designed to guide clinical practice.
  3. Cost-benefit analyses describe the costs and benefits of an intervention to determine whether the benefit of the intervention is worth the cost. Includes both financial costs and patient productivity potential.
  4. Evidence summary is a single conclusion/summarization and synthesis of the knowledge gained from a review of research studies obtained through a scientific, rigorous approach. It is an all-inclusive term for a systematic review (Polit & Beck, 2012).
  5. Evidence-based practice.
     a. The conscientious, explicit, judicious use of current best evidence in making decisions about patient care (Fawcett & Garity, 2009).
     b. A problem-solving approach to clinical practice.
  6. Review of the literature.
     a. Single studies.
        (1) Experimental.
        (2) Quasi-experimental.
        (3) Nonexperimental.
        (4) Qualitative designs.
     b. Summaries of multiple research studies.
        (1) Systematic reviews with or without meta-analysis.
        (2) Systematic reviews with or without metasynthesis.
  7. Systematic review is a review of research evidence related to a specific clinical question (uses reproducible search strategies and rigorous appraisal methods) (Polit & Beck, 2012).
  8. Meta-analysis is a research technique that synthesizes and analyzes quantitative scientific evidence (includes experimental and quasi-experimental designs) (Polit & Beck, 2012).

9. Meta-synthesis is a research technique that synthesizes and analyzes qualitative scientific evidence (identified metaphors and concepts) (Polit & Beck, 2012).
10. A randomized control trial (RCT) is the random assignment of two of more groups, one to a treatment or other strategy (e.g., diagnostic procedure) and the other to a placebo or another type of strategy. A comparison of outcomes is then made between the groups (Polit & Beck, 2012).
11. An experimental design includes an intervention, control group, random assignment to the control or intervention group, and manipulation of an independent variable (Polit & Beck, 2012).
12. A quasi-experimental design includes an intervention, may have a control group, lacks random assignment, and has some manipulation of an independent variable (Polit & Beck, 2012).
13. A nonexperimental design may have an intervention, no random assignment, no control group, and no manipulation of an independent variable.
14. A qualitative study has no randomization, no manipulation of an independent variable, and little control over the natural environment (Polit & Beck, 2012).
15. Validity is reference made to a study's results and findings that have been obtained by sound scientific methods (Polit & Beck, 2012).
16. Reliability is a reference made to a study's effects on practice regarding consistency and dependability (Polit & Beck, 2012).
17. Research utilization is applying knowledge gained from a single research study or studies within the practice setting (Polit & Beck, 2012).

II. Gathering the EBP evidence to incorporate into practice.

A. Identifying the clinical practice problem.
   1. Establish consensus of nursing staff and interprofessional colleagues.
   2. Establish concensus of the clinical practice problem with patients and stakeholders.
   3. Investigate internal data, reports, and findings.

B. Identifying the right databases (Dearholt & Dang, 2012).
   1. Types of databases.
      a. Bibliographic database describes the article in an abstract or synopsis. The title, author, journal name, and publisher are provided.
      b. Full-text database provides the full text of the article as well as the abstract, title, author, journal name, publisher, and citations.
   2. Systematic approach to using appropriate literature (Facchaiano & Snyder, 2012).
      a. Determine the quality of the study.
      b. Identify the findings/results of the study.
      c. Consider how to put the evidence into practice.
      d. Obtain organizational support to implement findings.
      e. Initiate, monitor, and evaluate changes.
   3. Quantitative vs. qualitative research.
      a. Quantitative data is collected in numeric form, then statistical analyses are conducted (Polit & Beck, 2012). Consideration for use in practice should include evaluation of the:
         (1) Validity and reliability of the results.
         (2) Application of the results to one's personal clinical practice.
         (3) Reason for the study.
         (4) Decision for the sample size.
         (5) Validity and reliability of the instruments.
         (6) Data analysis.
         (7) Limitations or unusual occurrences during the study.
         (8) Congruency of the results with previous research.
      b. Qualitative data is collected in nonnumeric form through the use of methods such as interviews (indepth interviews, focus groups), journals, photographs, observations (participant observations, naturalistic observations, field experiments), life histories, and documents (Polit & Beck, 2012). Consideration for use in practice should include evaluation of the:
         (1) Credibility (validity) or rigor (reliability) of the results.
         (2) Interpretation of the human experience (conscious lived experience as seen by the individual [phenomenology] or group/cultural experience by the researcher immersing oneself [ethnography]).
         (3) Application of the results to one's personal clinical practice.
         (4) Reason for the study with the approach fitting the purpose.
         (5) Selection of study participants.
         (6) Techniques for the data collection and analysis.
         (7) Congruency of the results with previous research.
   4. Guideline databases. Locating guidelines is an important step in the process. Three specific concerns should guide the user:
      a. Validity of the recommendations.
      b. Identification of the recommendations.
      c. The usefulness of the recommendations. (See Table 2.1 for sample guidelines.)

Table 2.1

Suggested Guideline Databases

Source	Web Site
National Guideline Clearinghouse (NGC)	http://www.guideline.gov
CMA InfoBase	https://www.cma.ca/En/Pages/clinical-practice-guidelines.aspx
Health Services/Technology Assessment Text (HSTAT)	http://hstat.nlm.nih.gov
Guidelines Advisory Committee (GAC)	http://www.gacguidelines.ca
Scottish Intercollegiate Guideline Network (SIGN)	http://www.sign.ac.uk/guidelines/index.html
National Institute for Clinical Excellence (NICE)	http://www.nice.org.uk
Guidelines International Network (G-I-N)	http://www.G-I-N.net
American College of Physicians (ACP)	http://www.acponline.org/clinical/guidelines
American Academy of Pediatrics (AAP)	http://www.aap.org/en-us/professional-resources/practice-support/quality-improvement/Pages/Guidelines-and-Policy-Development.aspx
American Nephrology Nurses' Association (ANNA) Standards of Practice	https://www.annanurse.org/clinical-practice/practice/standards-practice
National Kidney Foundation KDOQI Guidelines	https://www.kidney.org/professionals/KDOQI/guidelines

C. Steps toward EBP (Melnyk & Fineout-Overholt, 2011).
1. Identify the clinical question.
   a. A focused clinical question is the driving force of the steps that follow in the EBP process.
   b. Form question in PICOT format.
      (1) P = patient population information, setting, or disorder; includes age, gender, and ethnicity as well as specification of disorder of concern.
      (2) I = intervention of interest: exposure to disease, diagnostic factors, risk behaviors.
      (3) C = comparison against something else: treatment medication vs. placebo, new intervention against the standard of care.
      (4) O = identification of an outcome variable.
      (5) T = time during which populations are observed for the outcome to occur.
2. Find the best evidence to answer the question.
   a. Determine the review criteria to select only those research studies that will answer the question. While there are numerous scales for levels of evidence, there is a lack of standardization of the definitions. Some scales use 3 levels others use 7 (ANA, 2014). See Table 2.2.
   b. Select appropriate searchable databases (see II. A. Identifying the right databases).
   c. Understand setup of the database to specify the search.
   d. Use database language to search. Put in appropriate symbols, words, combination of words, spacing, etc., to obtain information being requested.
3. Appraise the evidence.
   a. Does the study demonstrate validity?
   b. Determine if the results are reliable by assessing the size (number of participants) and the strength of the effect (difference between groups).
   c. Are the results applicable to the current clinical issue or question, and do they facilitate patient care?
4. Integrate the evidence into clinical practice, taking into account the current condition of the patient, resources available, clinician expertise, and patient preference and values.
5. Evaluate the changes and outcomes as a result of evidence implementation.

III. Barriers to incorporating evidence into practice
(Dearholt & Dang, 2012; Melnyk &Fineout-Overholt, 2011).

A. Individual limitations.
1. Lack of skills finding and then perusing databases.
2. Knowledge deficit regarding critiquing the quality of research.
3. Overwhelming experience to review the evidence.

Table 2.2

Rating the Strength of Evidence

Level 1	The highest level includes experimental studies in which the study participants are randomly assigned (by chance) to the treatment group or the control group. Also included in this level is meta-analysis of multiple randomized control trials. In this situation the results of similar research studies are pooled, quantitatively synthesized, and analyzed.
Level 2	Includes quasi-experimental studies in which there is manipulation of an independent variable, but no randomization or control group.
Level 3	Includes nonexperimental studies where there is no manipulation of the independent variable. These studies can be thought of as descriptive, comparative, or relational. Level 3 also includes qualitative studies that are explorative in nature – interviews, observations, focus groups. This level is the starting point for areas where little research exists. Meta-synthesis is used to critically analyze and synthesize the results of qualitative research in order to interpret and translate findings of similar studies.

Source: The Johns Hopkins Hospital/The Johns Hopkins University as found on the American Nurses Association website: http://www.nursingworld.org. *Note*: The ANA's website contains a plethora of valuable information that can be accessed by members as well as nonmembers. The information can be located under "nursing research."

4. Unsure how to move from evidence to practice (e.g., changing policies and procedures, educational materials, or communications with clinical staff and patients).
5. Negative attitude toward research.

B. Organizational characteristics.
1. Dedicated time unavailable to find evidence.
2. Inadequate access to databases.
3. Lack of leadership support, incentives, and peer pressure.

IV. Facilitating EBP.

A. Identify clinical problem or challenge.
1. Prioritize clinical issues or problems.
2. Use internal clinical data to support issue.
3. Interview patient populations potentially at risk.
4. Review facility policies and procedures, as appropriate.

B. Promote a culture of organizational acceptance for EBP (see Table 2.3).
1. Transferability.
2. Feasibility.
3. Cost-benefit ratio.

C. Incorporate research findings into practice.
1. Revise facility policies and procedures, protocols, educational materials as needed while incorporating health care staff and patient feedback.
2. Educate staff and interprofessional colleagues impacted by the change.
3. Establish a launch date for the clinical practice change.
4. Evaluate and continuously monitor the impact of the clinical change. Refine as needed.

D. Promote acceptance among colleagues (Melnyk & Fineout-Overholt, 2011).
1. Assess with surveys and focus groups.
2. Identify baseline knowledge.
3. Identify real case scenarios and how EBP would address the situations better.

SECTION B
Standards for Care
Lisa Micklos

I. Standards.

A. Definition: authoritative statements defined and promoted by the profession by which the quality of practice, service, or education can be evaluated (ANA, 2010).

B. History: Since 1976, the American Nurses Association (ANA) has collaborated with nursing specialty practice organizations to develop and publish the standards of nursing practice, and later to incorporate the scope of specialty practice.
1. Development process led by ANA; specialty nursing organizations and others are included in draft development and review.
2. Final standards reviewed and adopted independently by individual specialty nursing organizations.

Table 2.3

Factors to Consider When Evaluating the Results of a Research Study that Could Potentially Change Practice in a Facility

Key team members should evaluate a research article and decide if a change in practice is indicated.	
Step 1	The first thing to consider is whether or not the study under review applies to the particular patient population. If not, go no further.
Step 2	Critique the research article. a. Does the title correctly portray the article? b. Is there an abstract that appropriately describes the article? c. Does the introduction describe the purpose of the study? d. Is the problem clearly stated? e. Is the purpose of performing the study well-defined? f. Is the research question(s) stated if applicable? g. Consider the theoretical framework of the study. h. Examine the literature review that should be relevant, comprehensive, and recent. It should support the need for performing the study. i. Scrutinize the methods employed by the study. Things to be considered include the research design, the sample size, the data collection tool, the way the data was collected, and the manner in which reliability and validity were addressed. j. Pour over the analysis of the data. Was the authors approach consistent with the study question(s) and the study's design? k. Review the discussion, the limitations, and the conclusion. l. Determine the level and quality of the evidence.
Step 3	Other factors to consider: feasibility (think about what would be required to make the change) and the cost/benefit ratio (carefully deliberate before taking the suggestion to administration).
Step 4	Make a team decision. Decisions based on evidence will promote organizational acceptance of change.

Adapted from Kaplan, L. (2014). *Framework for how to read and critique a research study*. American Nurses Association. http://www.nursingworld.org and Polit, D.F., & Beck, C.T. (2012). *Nursing research: Generating and assessing evidence for nursing practice* (9th ed.). Philadelphia: Wolters Kluwer, Lippincott Williams & Wilkins.

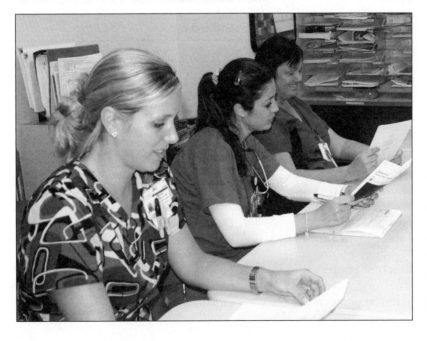

Key team members evaluate a research article and decide if a change in practice is indicated. If the study is not applicable to the particular patient population, they will go no further.

C. Purpose.
   1. Describes a competent level of nursing care (Standards of Practice) and a competent level of behavior in the professional role (Standards of Professional Performance).
   2. Describes the duties that all registered nurses, regardless of role, population, or specialty, are expected to perform competently.

D. Assumptions.
   1. Nursing practice is individualized to meet the unique needs of the health care consumer or situation.
   2. Caring is central to the practice of the registered nurse.
   3. Registered nurses use the nursing process to provide individualized care to those requiring nursing care.
   4. A positive correlation exists between the professional work environment and the registered nurse's ability to practice nursing.
   5. Standards are subject to change with the dynamics of the nursing profession as new practice and clinical evidence are developed.

II. Standards of Practice.

A. Describe a competent level of nursing care as demonstrated by the nursing process (ANA, 2010b).
   1. Assessment.
   2. Diagnosis.
   3. Outcomes identification.
   4. Planning.
   5. Implementation.
      a. Coordination of care.
      b. Health teaching and health promotion.
      c. Consultation.
      d. Prescriptive authority and treatment.
   6. Evaluation.

B. Provides a framework for nurse decision making.

C. Underlying assumptions that influence nursing practice.
   1. Provide age-appropriate and culturally and ethnically sensitive care.
   2. Maintain a safe environment.
   3. Educate patients.
   4. Assure continuity of care.
   5. Coordinate care across settings and among caregivers.
   6. Manage information.
   7. Communicate effectively.
   8. Use technology.

III. Standards of professional performance.

A. Describe a competent level of behavior in the professional role (ANA, 2010).
   1. Ethics.
   2. Education.
   3. Evidence-based practice and research.
   4. Quality of practice.
   5. Communication.
   6. Leadership.
   7. Collaboration.
   8. Professional practice evaluation.
   9. Resource utilization.
   10. Environmental health.

B. Expectation that nurses engage in professional role activities, including leadership, appropriate to their education and position.

C. Expectation that nurses are accountable for their professional actions to themselves, their health care consumers, their peers, and ultimately to society.

IV. Nephrology Nursing Guidelines.

A. Historical overview.
   1. 1972 – The American Association of Nephrology Nurses and Technicians (AANNT) published the first standards for hemodialysis.
   2. 1974 – The first issue of the *AANNT Journal* was published.
   3. 1975 – AANNT published *Standards of Clinical Practice for Transplantation*.
   4. 1977 – AANNT published *Standards of Clinical Practice for the Nephrology Patient*, which included hemodialysis, peritoneal dialysis, transplantation, and acute renal failure.
   5. 1982 – AANNT published *Nephrology Nursing Standards of Clinical Practice*. Revisions focused on the nursing process and expanded to include conservative management, hemoperfusion, and pediatrics.
   6. 1984 – *Nephrology Nursing Standards of Clinical Practice* reprinted without revision to reflect name change: *ANNA Standards of Clinical Practice*.
   7. 1988 – *ANNA Standards of Clinical Practice for Nephrology Nursing* were revised by the Clinical Practice Committee.
      a. Initiates concept of clinical problem or label.
      b. Introduces patient outcome statements.
      c. Acute patient included in each modality.
      d. Describes process as nursing management.
         (1) Assessment.
         (2) Intervention.
         (3) Patient teaching.
   8. 1993 – *Standards of Clinical Practice for Nephrology Nursing* (revision).

a. Introduced newly written standards of practice developed in collaboration with specialty nursing organizations and American Nurses Association.
b. Combined common clinical problems or labels into universal nursing standards of care.
c. Added:
(1) Therapeutic plasma exchange.
(2) Continuous renal replacement therapy (endorsed by the American Association of Critical Care Nurses).

9. 1999 – *ANNA Standards and Guidelines of Clinical Practice for Nephrology Nursing.*
a. Expanded edition included:
(1) Disease management.
(2) Pancreas transplantation.
(3) Sleep.
(4) Infection.
(5) Tuberculosis.
b. Updated standards of practice, including ANA's 1998 revision.
c. Introduced the concept of clinical practice guidelines by incorporating the National Kidney Foundation Kidney Disease Outcomes Quality Initiative (DOQI), 1997 CPG for anemia, adequacy of hemodialysis, adequacy of peritoneal dialysis, and vascular access.

10. 2002 – Advanced Practice Nurse Standards of Professional Performance.
a. Focus on professional performance.
b. Used ANA's *Scope of Practice and Standards of Advanced Practice Registered Nursing.*

11. 2005 – *Nephrology Nursing Standards of Practice and Guidelines for Care.*
a. Updated standards of practice, adapting ANA's 2004 revision; additional standards introduced.
(1) Coordination of care.
(2) Health teaching and health promotion.
(3) Consultation.
(4) Prescriptive authority and treatment.
(5) Leadership.
b. Added sections pertaining to the advanced practice nurse and the nephrology nursing role specialty.
c. Expanded universal guidelines for care by incorporating clinical practice guidelines from National Kidney Foundation Disease Outcomes Quality Initiative (NKF KDOQI), American Heart Association, American Diabetes Association, and others.
(1) Nutrition and metabolic control.
(2) Dyslipidemia and reduction of cardiovascular disease risk factors.
(3) Hypertension.
(4) Sleep.
(5) Bone metabolism and disease.
d. Added new nephrology nursing care guidelines.
(1) Chronic kidney disease, stages 1 to 4.
(2) Self-care and home dialysis.
(3) Palliative care and end-of-life care.
(4) Self-management.
(5) Rehabilitation.

12. 2011 – *Nephrology Nursing Scope and Standards*, 7th edition (Gomez, 2011).
a. Defines nephrology nursing.
b. Reviews nursing theorists.
c. Describes the evolution of nephrology nursing.
d. Integrates "how to use" tools such as clinical vignettes.

B. Definition. Nephrology nursing guidelines for care incorporate, when available, evidence-supported recommendations or interdisciplinary clinical practice guidelines from NKF-KDOQI, American Heart Association, American Diabetes Association, Centers for Disease Control, Association for the Advancement of Medical Instrumentation, Renal Physicians Association, International Society for Peritoneal Dialysis (ISPD), and others. For the most part, the nephrology nursing guidelines are lacking a strong body of supporting evidence and are dependent upon expert clinical opinion.

C. Purpose.
1. Statements that include recommendations to optimize patient care.
2. Provides direction for professional practice and a framework for the evaluation of the professional nurse.

SECTION C
The National Kidney Foundation Disease Outcomes Quality Initiative and The Kidney Disease Improving Global Outcomes

M. Sue McManus

I. Definition.

A. The National Kidney Foundation Kidney Disease Outcomes Quality Initiative (KDOQI) guidelines provide clinical practice guidelines to improve outcomes in individuals across the stages of kidney disease (NKF, 2013a).

B. The Kidney Disease: Improving Global Outcomes (KDIGO) is a global nonprofit organization governed by an international board and managed by the National Kidney Foundation (Kidney Disease: Improving Global Outcomes (KDIGO) (NKF, 2013a; NKF, 2013c).

C. KDIGO provides global clinical practice guidelines and promotes implementation of those guidelines to improve the care and outcomes of patients with kidney disease worldwide (KDIGO, 2013a; NKF, 2013c).

D. The KDOQI and KDIGO provide evidence-based information to aid in clinical decision making (KDIGO, 2013a; NKF, 2013a).

E. The KDOQI and KDIGO guidelines are not standards of care (KDIGO, 2013a; NKF, 2012).

II. History of KDOQI.

A. Dialysis Outcomes Quality Initiative (DOQI) (NKF, 2013b).
   1. The initiative began in 1995.
   2. The initial focus was only on patients on dialysis.
   3. The first guidelines were released in 1997.

B. The Kidney Disease Outcomes Quality Initiative (KDOQI) (NKF, 2013b).
   1. The scope of the initiative changed in 1999.
   2. The name changed from DOQI to KDOQI.
   3. The focus changed to include all stages of chronic kidney disease.
      a. Goals to define and classify stages of chronic kidney disease.
         (1) Prevent loss of kidney function.
         (2) Slow progression to kidney failure.
         (3) Lessen organ dysfunction and comorbid condition in those individuals with chronic kidney failure.

III. Development of the KDOQI guidelines (NKF, 2013a).

A. Development of each guideline takes 2 to 3 years.

B. Members of multidisciplinary work groups are chosen based on leadership, commitment to quality care, and clinical expertise.

C. Each work group critically reviews the available literature using the approach based on the Agency for Healthcare Research and Quality procedure.

D. The rationale and evidence for the guidelines are provided.

E. Each guideline has a time for open review before publication.

F. Comments provided during the open review are considered by each work group.

G. Final guidelines are published.

H. Updates are considered 3 years after publication if a sufficient body of evidence is available.

I. Updates undergo the same development process, but it takes 1 to 2 years to publish an updated guideline.

J. Guidelines have been translated into more than a dozen languages.

K. Guidelines have provided the basis of clinical performance measures developed and put into effect by the Centers for Medicare and Medicaid Services (CMS) (NKF, 2013b).

IV. Components of the KDOQI guidelines (NKF, 2006a).

A. Introduction.
B. Summary.
C. Introduction and rationale.
D. Process and methods.
E. Guideline statements.
F. Rationale statements.
G. Evidence base for the guidelines.
H. Tables of the evidence.
I. Limitations of the current guidelines.
J. Clinical considerations.
K. Recommendations for research.
L. Guidelines that could be used to assess clinical performance.

V. Current guidelines (NKF, 2013a).

A. Most KDOQI guidelines are available on the Web.

B. KDOQI guidelines are kept in dialysis units and clinics.

C. To date, 13 KDOQI guidelines have been developed for patients with kidney disease.

D. Expert workgroups update existing guidelines when the body of evidence indicates important changes.

E. Published guidelines and the website for each are located in the reference list.
   1. Guidelines for Dialysis Care.
      a. Hemodialysis Adequacy (NKF, 2006a).
      b. Peritoneal Dialysis Adequacy (NKF, 2006a).
      c. Vascular Access (NKF, 2006a).
      d. Cardiovascular Disease in Dialysis Patients (NKF, 2005b).
   2 Guidelines for CKD Care.
      a. Update of the Diabetes and Chronic Kidney Disease (NKF, 2012).

b. Diabetes and Chronic Kidney Disease (NKF, 2007b).
c. Anemia in Chronic Kidney Disease (NKF, 2006b).
d. 2007 Anemia in Chronic Kidney Disease – Update of Hemoglobin Target (NKF, 2007a).
e. Chronic Kidney Disease: Evaluation, Classification, and Stratification (NKF, 2002).
f. Bone Metabolism and Disease in Chronic Kidney Disease (NKF, 2003a).
g. Bone Metabolism and Disease in Children with Chronic Kidney Disease (NKF, 2005a).
h. Hypertension and Antihypertensive Agents in Chronic Kidney Disease (NKF, 2004a).
i. Managing Dyslipidemia in Chronic Kidney Disease (NKF, 2004b).
j. Nutrition in Children with CKD: 2008 Update (NKF, 2009).
k. Nutrition in Chronic Renal Failure (NKF, 2000).

VI. NKF Commentaries on KDIGO Guidelines (NKF, 2013a).

A. KDOQI workgroup of U.S. experts review KDIGO guidelines.

B. Write and publish commentary regarding local applicability and importance.

C. Form basis for U.S. specific implementation tools produced under KDOQI brand.

D. Current commentaries (NKF, 2013a).
   1. KDOQI US Commentary on the 2012 KDIGO Clinical Practice Guideline for Glomerulonephritis.
   2. KDOQI US Commentary on the 2012 KDIGO Clinical Practice Guideline for Anemia in CKD.
   3. KDOQI US Commentary on the 2012 KDIGO Clinical Practice Guideline for Management of Blood Pressure in CKD.
   4. KDOQI Acute Kidney Injury Commentary.
   5. KDOQI Hepatitis C Commentary.
   6. KDOQI Mineral and Bone Disorder (CKD-MBD) Commentary.
   7. KDOQI Commentary on Care of the Kidney Transplant Patient.

VII. Use of KDOQI in practice.

A. Use KDOQI guidelines to make informed decisions about managing CKD patients at specific stages of the disease process.

B. Use KDOQI guidelines in assessment of CKD patient with comorbid conditions.

C. Use KDOQI guidelines to translate complexities of CKD stages and interventions.

D. Use KDOQI guidelines in context of caring and respect for patients and their families.

E. Use KDOQI guidelines with consideration for age, gender, environment, and cultural sensitivity.

VIII. History of KDIGO (KDIGO, 2013a).

A. Global nonprofit foundation established 2003.

B. Governed by international board.

C. Managed by National Kidney Foundation.

IX. Development of KDIGO Guidelines (KDIGO, 2013c).

A. Topic selection and prioritization criteria.

B. KDIGO hosted international Controversies Conferences.

C. International multidisciplinary work group selection.

D. Evidence review team contracted to align methods used by the Evidence-Based Practice Center Program of the Agency for Health Care Research and Quality.

E. Guideline development process by work group over course of 1 to 2 years.

F. Evidence rating according to Grades of Recommendation, Assessment, Development, and Evaluation (GRADE) methodology.

G. Public review inviting feedback.

H. Publication.

I. Dissemination and implementation via Implementation Task Force.

J. Updating existing KDIGO guidelines for credibility.

X. Components of KDIGO Guidelines (KDIGO, 2013b).

A. Introduction.
B. Methodological approach.
C. Recommendations.
D. Rationale.
E. Background.
F. Limitations of current sources.
G. Evaluation and treatment.
H. Summary and research recommendations.

XI. Current KDIGO Guidelines (KDIGO, 2013b).

Each guideline is available as a PDF file at http://kdigo.org/home/guidelines

A. KDIGO 2012 Clinical Practice Guideline for the Evaluation and Management of Chronic Kidney Disease.

B. KDIGO Clinical Practice Guideline for the Management of Blood Pressure in Chronic Kidney Disease.

C. KDIGO Clinical Practice Guideline for Glomerulonephritis (GN).

D. KDIGO Clinical Practice Guideline for Acute Kidney Injury.

E. KDIGO Clinical Practice Guideline for Anemia in Chronic Kidney Disease.

F. KDIGO Guideline for Chronic Kidney Disease-Mineral and Bone Disorder.

G. KDIGO Guideline for Care of the Kidney Transplant Recipient.

H. KDIGO Guideline for the Prevention, Diagnosis, Evaluation, and Treatment of Hepatitis C in Chronic Kidney Disease.

XII. Use of KDIGO in practice.

A. Use KDIGO information to assist in decision making about managing CKD patients.

B. Use KDIGO guidelines, taking into account individual patient needs, resources available, and unique limitations of specific institution or practice.

C. Use KDIGO guidelines, taking into account the international stage for which they are written and the possible need to adapt to meet the needs of a specific patient population and health care system.

SECTION D
The Dialysis Outcomes and Practice Patterns Study

Caroline S. Counts

I. Overview.

A. The Dialysis Outcomes and Practice Patterns Study (DOPPS) began in 1996 as a prospective cohort study of hemodialysis practices.

B. The DOPPS projects are coordinated by research scientists and staff of Arbor Research Collaborative for Health located in Ann Arbor, Michigan.

C. A representative and random sample of patients from dialysis facilities located around the world allow data to be collected over time.

D. Differences in practice patterns are described and are correlated with differences in outcomes. Examples:
1. Staffing ratios and composition.
2. Size of the facility.
3. Information related to the vascular access used.
4. Dialysis prescription.
5. Dialysis delivery system.

E. Outcomes are defined as patient events associated with human and economic consequences. Examples:
1. Death.
2. Hospital admission.
3. Failure of vascular access.
4. Quality of life.
5. Development of new medical conditions.

F. The measured outcomes are adjusted for patient comorbidities.

G. Understanding factors associated with patient outcomes may improve patient care and lower mortality and morbidity rates.

II. The DOPPS practice monitor (DPM).

A. The DPM reports recent trends in hemodialysis practice in the United States following changes in payment and regulatory policies.

B. Observations can be made with data obtained from other DOPPS countries to determine if results are similar to those seen in the United States.

C. Details can be found on the DOPPS website regarding the most recent trends. In 2013, these included:
1. Anemia.
2. Mineral bone disorder (MBD).
3. Dialysis adequacy and dialysis session length.

D. Data can be browsed by clinical topic, facility, or patient characteristics.

III. The DOPPS annual reports.

A. Annual reports include more than a decade of descriptive statistics and demonstrate how the results are trending over time.

B. Provide country-specific results and trends. Data is reported from a variety of practice areas including:
   1. Anemia.
   2. Comorbidities.
   3. Demographics.
   4. Dialysis dose and treatments.
   5. Medications.
   6. Mineral metabolism.
   7. Nutrition.
   8. Quality of life.
   9. Vascular access.

C. Include a summary of the DOPPS study design and methods.

IV. Latest projects to emerge from the DOPPS.

A. The Peritoneal Dialysis Outcomes and Practice Patterns Study (PDOPPS).
   1. International study.
   2. Addresses areas of practice uncertainty.
   3. Pinpoints areas where research is needed.
   4. Proposed topics identified by the International Society for Peritoneal Dialysis and other leaders in peritoneal dialysis.

B. The Chronic Kidney Disease Outcomes and Practice Patterns Study (CKDOPPS).
   1. International study.
   2. Aims to provide reliable evidence focusing on:
      a. Treatment options and the impact on patient survival.
      b. Quality of life.
      c. Effects of delaying or avoiding the initiation of dialysis.
      d. Analysis of the costs associated with treatment.
   3. The intention is to identify the most successful treatment practices.

V. The DOPPS mission encourages sharing of information.

A. All information in this section was gleaned from the DOPPS website: http://www.dopps.org
   1. The website contains a wealth of information (data and graphics) that is available to interested individuals.
   2. Slides for public use may be downloaded and used as long as the source is properly cited.
   3. The DOPPS annual report is available online and may be downloaded if desired.

B. DOPPS investigators have published research papers that can be searched via the website.

C. The DOPPS provides additional methods of sharing information.
   1. Public teleconferences are held when the DPM releases major data. Details of upcoming teleconferences can be found at http://www.dopps.org/DPM/
   2. The home page of the DOPPS website allows anyone interested to sign up for the DOPPS e-newsletter: http://www.dopps.org

Section E
United States Renal Data System
Gail S. Wick

I. Definition.

A. The United States Renal Data System (USRDS) is an extensive national data system that collects, analyzes, and distributes information about end stage renal disease (ESRD) in the United States (USRDS, 2013).

B. Population covered includes Medicare and non-Medicare ESRD patients (USRDS, 2013).

C. Funded by the National Institute of Diabetes and Digestive and Kidney Diseases (NIDDK) in collaboration with the Centers for Medicare and Medicaid (CMS) (Health Indicators, 2014).

II. History (UM-KECC, n.d.).

A. Started in 1988 in Washington, DC, by Friedrich K. Port, Robert A. Wolfe, and Philip J. Held, with a NIH/NIDDK grant.

B. In 1993, the second USRDS contract was awarded to the same team, but at the University of Michigan.

C. The grant is renewed periodically.

D. USRDS Coordinating Center, 1415 Washington Heights, Suites 3645 SPH I, Ann Arbor, MI 48109.

III. Purpose (USRDS, 2013).

A. To collect, analyze, and distribute accurate data about ESRD in the United States.
   1. Annual Data Report (ADR) on ESRD and CKD in the United States.
   2. Fulfillment of data requests.
   3. Presentation of its research results at national conferences and in peer-reviewed journals.

B. USRDS data.
   1. Data include demographic, treatment, and

transplant data, as well as data from special studies done by the USRDS.
2. Data sources: CMS's Renal Management Information System (REMIS), Medical Evidence Form (CMS-2728), ESRD Death Notification Form (CMS-2746), UNOS transplant and wait-list data, and other CMS data supplements.
3. Data availability – 1988 to present.

C. Data are public domain.

D. Works closely with members of CMS, the United States Network for Organ Sharing (UNOS), and the ESRD networks to achieve goals.

IV. Goals (Health Indicators, 2014; USRDS, 2013).

A. To characterize the ESRD population.

B. To determine the prevalence and incidence, along with trends in mortality and disease rates.

C. To investigate relationships among patient demographics, treatment modalities, and morbidity.

D. To report the cost of ESRD treatments and total burden of the program in the United States.

E. To identify new areas for special renal studies and support investigator-initiated research.

F. To provision data to support research.

V. Governance (USRDS, 2013).

A. The USRDS Coordinating Center provides administrative oversight.

B. The governing body of the USRDS is the Steering Committee.
1. Coordinates activities among the centers.
2. Assures data availability.
3. Provides oversight of the production of the Annual Data Report.

C. Committees within the USRDS.
1. USRDS External Expert Committee.
   a. Advises on appropriate and special studies, data studies, and analyses.
   b. Reviews annual data reports and manuscripts.
2. Data Management Advisory committee (DMAC).
   a. Composition: members from CMS, Network Forum representatives, database technical staff, and appointees.
   b. Addresses the accuracy and completeness of the data provided to USRDS.
   c. Ensures timely fulfillment of data requests.
3. Annual Data Report Committee (ADRC).
   a. Reviews past data reports (ADRs) and proposals for future editions.
   b. Reviews ideas for expanded date availability on USRDS website.
4. Information Systems Committee (ISC).
   a. Reviews planned hardware requirements, systems configuration, documentation, and performance.
   b. Evaluates new technologies that may enhance the structure, function, and management of the database.
5. Special Studies Review and Implementation Committee (SSRIC).
   a. Serves as the operations committee for SSC proposals.
   b. Projects support of CC projects.
   c. Is a collaboration of CMS, the ESRD Networks, and providers.
6. Data Request Review Committee (DRRC).
   a. Reviews lengthy data requests.
   b. Makes recommendations to the Project Officers.
7. Renal Community Council (RCC).
   a. Composed of 30 professional, scientific, and advocacy groups interested in ESRD.
   b. Serves as liaison between USRDS and the ESRD community.

VI. USRDS Annual Report (USRDS, 2013).

A. Content provides valuable information for clinical care and quality purposes, research, and policy making.

B. Two volumes formatted as discussion, data tables, and raw data.

C. Content sample from Volume I in a typical annual report.
1. Overview of CKD in the United States.
2. CKD in the general population.
3. Morbidity and mortality in CKD.
4. Cardiovascular disease in CKD.
5. Prescription drug coverage in CKD.
6. Acute kidney injury.
7. Cost of CKD.
8. Reference tables – CKD.
9. Volume I highlights.

D. Content sample from Volume II from each annual report.
1. Introduction to ESRD in the United States.
2. Healthy people 2020.
3. Incidence, prevalence, patient characteristics, and treatment modalities.
4. Clinical indicators and preventive care.

5. Hospitalization.
6. Cardiovascular disease.
7. Mortality.
8. Part D prescription drug coverage in ESRD.
9. Transplantation.
10. Pediatric ESRD.
11. Special studies – rehabilitation, quality of life, and nutrition.
12. ESRD providers.
13. Cost of ESRD.
14. International comparisons.
15. Reference tables – ESRD.

E. Finding data on the website.
   1. Annual Data Report chapters address data trends on specific topics. The report is divided into two parts:
      a. Atlas section displays data using charts and graphs.
      b. Reference tables are devoted to the ESRD population.
   2. Choose Atlas or Reference Tables from the USRDS home page: http://www.usrds.org
   3. Data from previous years are available.
   4. Analysis files are available to researchers with approved research proposals.

VII. Contacting USRDS and accessing information.

A. Mailing address:
USRDS Coordinating Center, 1415 Washington Heights, Suite 3645 SPH I | Ann Arbor, MI 48109

B. Phone: 1-888-99USRDS or 734-763-7793

C. Email: usrds@usrds.org

D. Website: http://www.usrds.org

SECTION F

Consolidated Renal Operations in a Web-enabled Network

Alicia M. Horkan

I. Introduction.

A. United States Renal Data System's (USRDS) Annual Data Report (2012) stated there were greater than 590,000 dialysis modality and transplant patients treated for end-stage renal disease (ESRD) in 2010.

B. The number of dialysis and transplant patients treated for ESRD continues to increase by 3–4% each year (Delva, 2013).

C. At the end of 2010, patients with ESRD were being treated at more than 5,800 Medicare certified facilities nationwide (Delva, 2013).

D. Centers for Medicare & Medicaid Services (CMS) recognized the need to streamline the data submission process by facilities treating individuals with ESRD (Delva, 2013).

II. Definition. CROWNWeb is a secure Internet-based data collection system developed by CMS to facilitate facility electronic submission of patient data (Delva, 2013).

III. History.

A. Data monitoring by CMS has been difficult because of the large number of individuals receiving treatment for ESRD (Delva, 2013).
   1. Individual facilities traditionally maintained facility data and shared the data with CMS and ESRD networks when requested.
   2. Paper submissions of data for a selected 5–8% of the dialysis population limited the ability of CMS to adequately monitor trends for quality improvement initiatives.

B. In an effort to improve efficacy of data collection, in 2008, CMS began development of a secure, electronic data collection system identified as CROWNWeb (Delva, 2013).
   1. An announcement was made by CMS in Conditions for Coverage (CfC) for ESRD facilities describing the development and release of CROWNWeb.

C. In 2009, CROWNWeb was released to select ESRD facilities to begin secure submission of and access to patient data (Delva, 2011).
   1. Since the initial release, two phase-in releases were implemented in anticipation of national release in 2012.
   2. Feedback from initial and phase-in facilities was used to make improvements to enhance the program prior to national release.

D. In June 2012, CROWNWeb was released for use by all ESRD facilities (Delva, 2013).
   1. Electronic submission replaced mailed paper submission to ESRD networks.
   2. Data submitted is used by CMS to support quality improvement initiatives.

E. Since release, CROWNWeb has been used by more than 15,000 registered users at CMS certified ESRD facilities (Delva, 2013).

F. System updates occur as needed integrating feedback from users to assist facilities in meeting CMS submission requirements (Delva, 2013).

IV. Purpose.

A. CROWNWeb was developed and implemented to aid dialysis facilities meeting CMS Conditions for Coverage (CfC) (2008) Section 494.180 (h) which stated Medicare-certified dialysis facilities must submit patient and facility data electronically (Delva, 2011).

B. Data for 100% of the ESRD population provides a more accurate picture of the entire dialysis population (Delva, 2011).

C. CROWNWeb facilitates timely, accurate, and efficient use of patient data by CMS (Delva 2013).

V. Goals.

A. CROWNWeb will support collection of complete and high quality patient and facility data (Delva, 2011).

B. ESRD population will experience increased benefits through use of health information technology (Delva, 2011).

C. CMS will be equipped with accurate data to better analyze the health status of the ESRD community (Delva, 2011).

D. Data collected and submitted through CROWNWeb will support CMS Quality Incentive Program (QIP) (Delva, 2011).

VI. Use by dialysis providers.

A. Project CROWNWeb provides online training for all staff members using the CROWNWeb system at all Medicare-certified dialysis centers.
   1. Training modules are task-specific to promote staff competence with each component of the CROWNWeb system.
   2. Staff members involved in accessing and entering data in CROWNWeb create a Learning Management System (LMS) account on the Project CROWNWeb internet site that is used to access the free training modules.
   3. Designated user roles for CROWNWeb are facility administrator, facility editor, and facility viewer.
      a. Facility administrator.
      b. Facility editor.
      c. Facility viewer.

B. Various types of patient data are submitted by ESRD facilities.
   1. Patient admission and discharge history.
   2. CMS-2728 form: ESRD Medical Evidence Report: Medical entitlement and/or patient registration.
   3. CMS-2746 form: Death Notification.
   4. CMS-2744 form: Facility Survey.
   5. Patient Attributes and Related Treatment (PART).
   6. Clinical values for hemodialysis, peritoneal dialysis, and vascular access.

C. Reports.
   1. CROWNWeb is designed to allow individual ESRD facilities to run reports that permit monitoring and trending of patient and facility data.
      a. Vascular access report.
      b. Clinical data report.

SECTION G
United Network for Organ Sharing
Linda S. Wright

I. Definition.

A. The United Network for Organ Sharing (UNOS) is a private, nonprofit organization that coordinates the U.S. organ transplant system(UNOS, n.d.-a).

B. Contracted by the federal government (UNOS, n.d.-a).

C. Five classes of members (UNOS, 2009).
   1. Institutional members.
      a. Organ procurement organizations.
      b. Transplant centers.
      c. Histocompatibility laboratory serving at least one transplant center.
   2. Medical/scientific members: established nonprofit organization with an interest in organ donation and/or transplantation.
      a. Medical or scientific professional organization.
      b. Membership includes professional involved in organ transplantation.
      c. Other organization(s) with letters of recommendation from at least three organizations that meet the criteria for Institutional Membership.
   3. Public organization members: established nonprofit organization with an interest in organ donation and/or transplantation.
      a. Organization involved in organ donation.
      b. Organization providing support or services to

transplant candidates and/or recipients, or their families.
   c. Hospital that has referred at least one potential organ or tissue donor per year.
   d. Other organization(s) with letters of recommendation from at least three organizations that meet the criteria for membership in any class other than Individual Member.
4. Business members.
   a. Established organization with an interest in organ donation and/or transplantation.
   b. Commercial relationship with at least two active Institutional Members.
5. Individual members: person with interest or expertise in organ donation and/or transplantation.
   a. Present/former members of the UNOS Board of Directors or a UNOS Committee.
   b. Transplant candidates.
   c. Transplant recipients.
   d. Organ/tissue donors.
   e. Family members of transplant candidates/recipients or organ/tissue donors.
   f. Present/former employees or contractors for organ procurement organizations, transplant centers, or histocompatibility laboratories.
   g. Former employees of government agencies involved in donation and/or transplantation who demonstrate a continued interest and involvement.
   h. Other individuals with interest and involvement in organ donation and/or transplantation, with letters of recommendation from at least three people, each of whom must meet the criteria for Individual Membership.

II. History.

A. Uniform Anatomical Gift Act (National Conference of Commissioners on Uniform State Laws, 1968).
   1. Originally enacted in 1968.
   2. Standardized state laws concerning donation of organs and tissues from deceased (cadaveric) donors.
   3. Encouraged anatomical gifts, and facilitated transplantation and other therapies that use donated organs and tissues.

B. South-Eastern Regional Organ Procurement Program (American Foundation for Donation & Transplant, n.d.; Petechuk, 2006).
   1. Founded in 1969 by two physicians from the Medical College of Virginia and Duke University.
      a. Realized that better tissue matching between kidney donors and recipients led to better transplant outcomes.
      b. Successfully experimented with sharing organs between hospitals.
      c. Developed a network of organ sharing and organ procurement among nine hospitals in four states, between Baltimore and Atlanta.
   2. Renamed South-Eastern Organ Procurement Foundation (SEOPF) in 1975 (Petechuk, 2006; UNOS, n.d.-c, n.d.-f).
      a. 18 charter hospitals in six states.
      b. Developed a national organ procurement and allocation system.
         (1) Computerized national wait list.
         (2) Computerized system for the cross-matching of donors and recipients.
            (a) Computer system called United Network for Organ Sharing (UNOS).
            (b) Developed in 1977.
         (3) 1982: Started the Kidney Center.
            (a) Staffed 24 hours/day.
            (b) For regional placement of organs.
   3. UNOS separated from SEOPF in 1984 (UNOS, n.d.-f).
      a. Independent nonprofit organization.
      b. Due to growing national demand for organ transplantation.

C. National Organ Transplant Act of 1984.
   1. Prohibited the purchase of human organs.
   2. Established Organ Procurement Organizations (OPO) for deceased donor transplants.
      a. Identify potential organ donors.
      b. Arrange for tissue typing of donated organs.
      c. Coordinate allocation, acquisition, preservation, and transportation of donated organs.
   3. Established the Organ Procurement and Transplantation Network (OPTN).
      a. Private, nonprofit organization.
      b. Facilitate recovery and placement of deceased donor organs.
      c. Maintain a registry of data regarding organ donation and transplantation.

D. UNOS was granted the first OPTN contract in 1986 by the U.S. Department of Health and Human Services (OPTN, n.d.-b; UNOS, n.d.-f).
   1. Contract has been renewed four times.
   2. UNOS remains the only organization ever to administer the OPTN.

III. Purpose (UNOS, n.d.-a, n.d.-b, n.d.-f).

A. Increase awareness of the need for donated organs and tissues.
   1. Active in state and national health community.
      a. Health fairs.

  b. Community events.
  c. Sporting events.
  d. Schools and universities.
  e. Staff and volunteers give presentations and distribute educational materials.
2. National Donor Memorial.
  a. Memorial garden and website.
  b. Designed by group of volunteers representing transplant recipients, live organ donors, and donor families.
  c. Honors eye, tissue, and organ donors in the United States.
3. Donate Life America.
  a. Founded by UNOS in 1992, but now an independent organization.
  b. Purpose is to inspire people to save and change lives through eye, tissue, and organ donation.

B. Maintain the national organ transplant waiting list. Secure Internet-based database (UNETSM) used to register potential transplant recipients.

C. Coordinate matching of deceased donor organs with potential recipients. Computer network (UNetSM) that links transplant centers and organ procurement organizations.
1. Accessible to transplant professionals 24 hours/day, 7 days/week.
2. Used to match organ donors with potential recipients.
3. Deceased donor organs are managed and offered using DonorNetSM.
  a. Integrated as part of the UNetSM computer network.
  b. Organs are able to be offered to all appropriate transplant centers simultaneously making organ matching and placement more efficient than in the past, when organ offers and the dissemination of clinical information had to be handled through multiple faxes and telephone calls.

D. Coordinate distribution and transportation of donated organs.

E. Collect and report data on organ donors, transplant recipients, and transplant outcomes.
1. UNetSM contains data regarding every solid organ donation and transplant performed in the United States since 1986.
2. UNETSM analyzes and publishes data related to the patient waiting list, organ matching, and transplants performed.
3. Data is available at the national, regional, state, and transplant center level.

F. Development of policies governing the allocation of donated organs.
1. Uses a collaborative process of policy development which encourages participation by all members of the transplant community, the public, and the government.
  a. Policy changes are recommended by a committee.
  b. A document is prepared and distributed for public comment that outlines the proposed policy change and the supporting rationale.
  c. The committee reviews the public comments and makes any appropriate change to the proposal.
  d. The committee adds their responses to the public comments, and makes their final recommendations to the Board of Directors, which votes on the proposed policy.
2. All policies must be reviewed and approved by the U.S. Department of Health and Human Services, and then becomes binding as federal regulation.

G. Establish training and experience criteria for transplant physicians and surgeons.

H. Development of professional education resources.

I. Education of the public with regard to organ transplantation.
1. Patient brochures and fact sheets.
  a. Transplantation and donation process.
  b. Living organ donation.
  c. National, regional, state, and transplant center-specific reports.
2. Transplant Living website: http://www.transplantliving.org

IV. Goals.

A. OPTN Primary Goals (OPTN, n.d.-a).
1. Increase the efficiency and effectiveness of organ sharing.
2. Increase fairness and equity within the organ allocation system.
3. Increase the number of organs that are available to be used for transplant.

B. OPTN Strategic Plan Goals (UNOS, 2013).
1. Increase the number of transplants performed.
2. Improve patient access to transplantation.
3 Improve the survival of patients with end-stage organ failure.
4. Improve patient safety with regard to transplantation.
5. Improve the safety of live organ/tissue donors.
6. Promote the efficient operation of the OPTN.

V. Governance.

A. Board of directors.
1. Establishes goals and policies (UNOS, 2009).
2. Consists of 41 elected members (OPTN, n.d.-c).
   a. 11 regional councilors.
   b. Transplant surgeons and physicians.
   c. Transplant coordinators.
   d. Histocompatibility professionals.
   e. Organ procurement organizations.
   f. Medical/scientific organizations.
   g. Members of the general public.
      (1) Transplant candidates and transplant recipients.
      (2) Live donors.
      (3) Donor family members.
      (4) Transplant recipient and candidate family members.

B. Permanent and ad hoc committees (OPTN, n.d.-d; UNOS, n.d.-f).
1. Ethics Committee.
   a. Deals with general ethical issues regarding procurement, allocation, distribution, and transplantation of organs.
   b. Does not address issues or disputes related to specific or individual patients.
   c. Makes recommendations to the board of directors regarding ethical issues within the national transplant network.
   d. Goal is to ensure that policies and activities are in keeping with accepted ethical standards.
2. Executive Committee.
   a. Reviews issues requiring the action or attention of the Board of Directors, and makes recommendations for action.
   b. Proposes resolution when conflicts exist between the recommendations of individual committees.
   c. Provides guidance concerning previous decisions and actions of the Board of Directors.
   d. Suspends or modifies the implementation of new policies that are not having the desired or expected effect.
3. Finance Committee.
4. Histocompatibility Committee.
   a. Reviews issues regarding histocompatibility testing, organ allocation, and laboratory and personnel qualifications.
   b. Goal is to promote patient safety, as well as improve patient outcomes and facilitate the best use of available organs.
5. Kidney Transplantation Committee.
   a. Reviews medical, scientific, and ethical issues with regard to the procurement, allocation, and distribution of kidneys.
   b. Considers both general implications and specific member issues regarding kidney transplant policies.
   c. Goal is the development of evidence-based policies.
      (1) Reducing the burden of CKD stage 5.
      (2) Increased utilization of donor kidneys.
      (3) Improving patient access to kidney transplantation.
      (4) Improving the health and outcomes of kidney transplant recipients.
6. Liver and Intestinal Organ Transplantation Committee.
   a. Reviews medical, scientific, and ethical issues with regard to the procurement, allocation, and distribution of liver and intestinal organs.
   b. Considers both general implications and specific member issues regarding liver and intestine transplant policies.
   c. Goal is the development of evidence-based policies.
      (1) Reducing the burden of liver disease.
      (2) Increasing utilization of donor organs.
      (3) Improving patient access to transplantation.
      (4) Improving the health and outcomes of transplant recipients.
7. Living Donor Committee.
   a. Develops policies regarding the donation and transplantation of live donor organs.
   b. Goal is to improve the informed decision making, safety, and follow-up of live organ donors.
8. Membership and Professional Standards Committee.
   a. Ensures that members meet criteria for membership.
      (1) Sets criteria for each class of membership.
      (2) Reviews applications for Institutional Membership and makes recommendations for action to the Board of Directors.
      (3) Reviews the performance, transplant activity, and outcomes of each transplant center.
      (4) Reviews all policy violations, and makes recommendations for action to the Board of Directors.
9. Minority Affairs Committee.
   a. Considers issues with regard to organ procurement, allocation, and transplant that have the potential to affect minority populations.
   b. Makes recommendations to the other committees and the Board of Directors to ensure that issues and/or needs of minority populations with regard to organ transplantation are addressed.

10. Operations and Safety Committee.
    a. Reviews near and actual adverse events regarding organ donation and transplantation, and identifies the need for changes in policy that will prevent similar future occurrences.
        (1) May recommend policy changes.
        (2) May recommend that they be made by another committee.
    b. Goal is to improve safety through the identification and correction of gaps in policies and procedures.
11. Organ Procurement Organization Committee.
    a. Considers issues pertaining to the organ procurement organizations as they work to increase the number of organs successfully and efficiently procured and transplanted.
    b. Considers the medical, scientific, and ethical issues related to the procurement of donated organs.
12. Pancreas Transplantation Committee.
    a. Reviews medical, scientific, and ethical issues with regard to the procurement, allocation, and distribution of pancreas organs and pancreas islet cells.
    b. Considers both general implications and specific member issues regarding pancreas and islet cell transplant policies.
    c. Goal is the development of evidence-based policies.
        (1) Reducing the burden of disease in recipients of, and candidates for, pancreas transplantation.
        (2) Increasing utilization of donor organs.
        (3) Improving patient access to pancreas transplantation.
        (4) Improving the health and outcomes of pancreas transplant recipients.
13. Patient Affairs Committee.
    a. Advises the Board of Directors and other committees with regard to the views of transplant patients and families concerning policies and other OPTN initiatives.
    b. Works alone or with other committees to develop initiatives or propose policies in areas of interest to transplant patients and families.
    c. Develops and makes recommendations concerning patient and family educational materials and information.
14. Pediatric Transplantation Committee.
    a. Considers medical, scientific, and ethical issues concerning organ procurement, allocation, and transplantation in the pediatric patient population.
        (1) Preoperative and postoperative issues.
        (2) Timely transplantation of pediatric patients.
        (3) Special needs of pediatric patients (medical, social, psychological).
    b. Goal is to develop evidence-based policies.
        (1) Improve access to transplantation.
        (2) Improve outcomes for all patients involved in transplantation in the pediatric population (including live donors and those on the waiting list).
15. Policy Oversight Committee.
    a. Reviews proposed and developing policies and gives recommendations to other committees and to the Board of Directors based on specific perspectives.
        (1) Degree to which proposals meet policy goals.
        (2) Whether or not proposals are adequately evidence-based.
    b. Goal is to ensure that OPTN initiatives are reviewed and evaluated in a standardized manner, and within the framework of the national system.
16. Thoracic Organ Transplantation Committee.
    a. Reviews medical, scientific, and ethical issues with regard to the procurement, allocation, and distribution of thoracic organs.
    b. Considers both general implications and specific member issues regarding heart and lung transplant policies.
    c. Goal is the development of evidence-based policies.
        (1) Reducing the burden of heart and lung disease.
        (2) Increasing utilization of donor thoracic organs.
        (3) Improving patient access to thoracic organ transplantation.
        (4) Improving the health and outcomes of the recipients of thoracic organ transplants.
17. Transplant Administrators Committee.
    a. Reviews issues concerning the administration of transplant programs.
    b. Provides input and makes recommendations to other committees and to the Board of Directors with regard to the potential impact on transplant program operations of developing policies and requirements.
    c. Develops tools to help facilitate the effective administration of transplant programs.
18. Transplant Coordinator Committee.
    a. Consists of transplant coordinators and procurement coordinators.
    b. Considers issues related to the organ procurement, allocation, and transplantation process.
    c. Considers the potential impact of proposed policies on procurement and transplant coordination.

(1) Education of transplant candidates, living donors, recipients, and families.
(2) Care of transplant candidates, living donors, recipients, and families.

d. Goal is improved quality, efficiency, and effectiveness of organ procurement and transplant coordination.

19. Ad Hoc Disease Transmission Advisory Committee.
a. Considers all issues regarding disease transmission through organ transplantation.
(1) Reviews individual cases to confirm disease transmission.
(2) Reviews combined data to determine the risk of donor-derived disease transmission.
b. Goal is to decrease donor-derived disease transmission through the education of members of the transplant community, as well as through the development of policies aimed at improving the safety of transplantation through the decrease of disease transmission.

20. Ad Hoc International Relations Committee.
a. Considers issues related to organ donors and transplant recipients that either come to or leave the country for transplant.
b. Considers general implications but may review specific cases.

C. Geographic Regions (UNOS, 2009).
1. 11 administrative regions.
2. Each region has a UNOS staff administrator for purposes of assisting with the coordination of regional activities.
3. Each region is represented on the Board of Directors, as well as on each standing committee, in order to assure geographic representation.

VI. Services (UNOS, n.d.-d, n.d.-e).

A. Research and technology.
1. PhD-level statisticians analyze clinical transplant data. Data is used to support policy decisions and evidence-based practice.
2. Research staff responds to more than 250 requests for transplantation data and analysis each month.

B. Conference planning.
1. Transplant Management Forum: annual national conference for transplant professionals.
a. Provides educational sessions.
b. Allows for networking opportunities.
2. UNOS Meeting Partners manage educational events for members of the transplant community.
a. Site selection and contract management.
b. Marketing.
c. Online registration.
d. Coordination of transportation and management of hotel logistics.
e. Management of exhibitors, speakers, and sponsors.

C. Advertisement. Transplant-related employment opportunities.

D. Education.
1. Center for Transplant System Excellence.
a. UNOS initiative to advance transplantation through the conducting of collaborative research and education.
b. Provides resources and leadership needed to facilitate ongoing multidisciplinary collaboration in the areas of evidence-based practice and clinical practice improvement.
c. Goals.
(1) Increase transplantation through a national system for paired kidney donation.
(2) Ensure that new research findings are applied to clinical practice through broadened clinical education.
(3) Facilitate research in areas of key importance to the advancement of organ transplantation.
2. Professional education.
a. Transplant Pro website: access to all UNOS member communications.
b. *UNOS Update*: bimonthly magazine.
c. Webinars for transplant professionals.
d. UNOS Primer.
(1) On-site conference.
(2) Information regarding UNOS structure, implementation of policy, compliance with policies, effective practice, and resources.
e. Policy brochures.
(1) Organ allocation.
(2) Listing at multiple transplant centers.
f. Data reports: national, regional, state, and transplant-center specific.

References

American Foundation for Donation and Transplant (AFDP). (n.d.). *Brief history*. Retrieved from http://www.seopf.org/intro.htm

American Nurses Association (ANA). (2010). *Nursing: Scope and standards of practice* (2nd ed.). Silver Spring, MD: Nursebooks.org.

Dearholt, S.L., & Dang, D. (2012). *John Hopkins nursing evidence-based practice: Model and guidelines* (2nd ed.), Indianapolis: Sigma Theta Tau International.

Delva, O. (2011). CROWNWeb update: Streamlining the future, exploring data submission solutions for the small provider. *Nephrology News & Issues, 25*(4), 26-27.

Delva, O. (2013). CROWNWeb: System enhancements, the ESRD QIP, and things to come. *Nephrology News & Issues, 27*(5), 30-32.

Dialysis Outcomes and Practice Patterns Study Program (DOPPS). (n.d.) http://www.dopps.org

Facchaiano, L., & Snyder, C.H. (2012). Evidence-based practice for the busy nurse practitioner: Part 2: Searching for the best evidence to clinical queries. *Journal of the American Academy of Nursing Practitioners*, 24, 640-648.

Fawcett, J., & Garity, J. (2009) *Evaluating research for evidence-based nursing practice*. Philadelphia: F.A. Davis Company.

Gomez, N. (Ed.). (2011). *Nephrology nursing scope and standards of practice* (7th ed.). Pitman, NJ: American Nephrology Nurses' Association.

Health Indicators Warehouse. (2014). *United States Renal Data System (USRDS)*. Retrieved from http://www.healthindicators.gov/Resources/DataSources/USRDS_163/Profile

Kidney Disease: Improving Global Outcomes (KDIGO). (2013a). *About us*. Retrieved from http://kdigo.org/home/about-us

Kidney Disease: Improving Global Outcomes (KDIGO). (2013b). *Clinical practice guidelines*. Retrieved from http://kdigo.org/home/guidelines

Kidney Disease: Improving Global Outcomes (KDIGO). (2013c). *Methods for development of KDIGO clinical practice guidelines*. Retrieved from http://kdigo.org/home/guidelines/development

Lee, M.C., Johnson, K.L., Newhouse, R.P., & Warren, J.I. (2013). Evidence-based practice process quality assessment: EPQA guidelines. *Worldview on Evidence-Based Nursing*, 10(3), 140-149.

Melnyk, B.M., & Fineout-Overholt, E. (2011). *Evidence-based practice in nursing & healthcare: A guide to best practice* (2nd ed.). Philadelphia: Wolters Kluwer, Lippincott Williams & Wilkins.

National Conference of Commissioners on Uniform State Laws. (1968). *Uniform Anatomical Gift Act*. Retrieved from http://www.uniformlaws.org/shared/docs/anatomical_gift/uaga%201968_scan.pdf

National Kidney Foundation (NKF). (2000). *Clinical practice guidelines for nutrition in chronic renal failure*. Retrieved from http://www.kidney.org/professionals/kdoqi/guidelines_updates/doqi_nut.html

National Kidney Foundation (NKF). (2002). *Clinical practice guidelines for chronic kidney disease: Evaluation, classification, and stratification*. Retrieved from http://www.kidney.org/professionals/kdoqi/guidelines_ckd/toc.htm

National Kidney Foundation (NKF). (2003a). *Clinical practice guidelines for bone metabolism and disease in chronic kidney disease*. Retrieved from http://www.kidney.org/professionals/kdoqi/guidelines_bone/index.htm

National Kidney Foundation (NKF). (2004a). *Clinical practice guidelines on hypertension and antihypertensive agents in chronic kidney disease*. Retrieved from http://www.kidney.org/professionals/kdoqi/guidelines_bp/index.htm

National Kidney Foundation (NKF). (2004b). *Clinical practice guidelines for managing dyslipidemia in chronic kidney disease*. Retrieved from http://www.kidney.org/professionals/KDOQI/guidelines_lipids/toc.htm

National Kidney Foundation (NKF). (2005a). *Clinical practice guidelines for bone metabolism and disease in children with chronic kidney disease*. Retrieved from http://www.kidney.org/professionals/kdoqi/guidelines_pedbone/index.htm

National Kidney Foundation (NKF). (2005b). *Clinical practice guidelines for cardiovascular disease in dialysis patients*. Retrieved from http://www.kidney.org/professionals/kdoqi/guidelines_cvd/index.htm

National Kidney Foundation (NKF). (2006a). *Clinical practice guidelines and clinical practice recommendations: 2006 updates – Hemodialysis adequacy, peritoneal dialysis adequacy, and vascular access*. Retrieved from http://www.kidney.org/professionals/KDOQI/guideline_upHD_PD_VA/index.htm

National Kidney Foundation (NKF). (2006b). *Clinical practice guidelines and clinical practice recommendations for anemia in chronic kidney disease*. Retrieved from http://www.kidney.org/professionals/kdoqi/guidelines_anemia/index.htm

National Kidney Foundation (NKF). (2007a). *Clinical practice guideline and clinical practice recommendations for anemia in CKD: 2007 update of hemoglobin target*. Retrieved from http://www.kidney.org/professionals/KDOQI/guidelines_anemiaUP/index.htm

National Kidney Foundation (NKF). (2007b). *Clinical practice guidelines and clinical practice recommendations for diabetes and chronic kidney disease*. Retrieved from http://www.kidney.org/professionals/KDOQI/guideline_diabetes

National Kidney Foundation (NKF). (2009). *Clinical practice guideline for nutrition in children with CKD: 2008 update*. Retrieved from http://www.kidney.org/professionals/KDOQI/guidelines_ped_ckd/index.htm

National Kidney Foundation (NKF). (2012). *Clinical practice guidelines and clinical practice recommendations for diabetes and CKD: 2012 update*. Retrieved from http://www.kidney.org/professionals/KDOQI/guidelines_diabetesUp/diabetes-ckd-update-2012.pdf

National Kidney Foundation (NKF). (2013a). *Guidelines and commentaries*. Retrieved from http://www.kidney.org/professionals/KDOQI/guidelines_commentaries.cfm

National Kidney Foundation (NKF). (2013b). *History*. Retrieved from http://www.kidney.org/about/history.cfm

National Kidney Foundation (NKF). (2013c). *Important milestones in NKF history*. Retrieved from http://www.kidney.org/about/milestones.cfm

National Organ Transplant Act, Pub. L. No. 98 Stat. 2339-2348 (1984).

Organ Procurement and Transplantation Network (OPTN). (n.d.-a). *About OPTN*. Retrieved from http://optn.transplant.hrsa.gov/optn

Organ Procurement and Transplantation Network (OPTN). (n.d.-b). *About OPTN: History*. Retrieved from http://optn.transplant.hrsa.gov/optn/history.asp

Organ Procurement and Transplantation Network (OPTN). (n.d.-c). *Board of directors Q&A*. Retrieved from http://optn.transplant.hrsa.gov/members/bodQA.asp

Organ Procurement and Transplantation Network (OPTN). (n.d.-d). *Members: Committees*. Retrieved from http://optn.transplant.hrsa.gov/converge/members/committees.asp

Petechuk, D. (2006). *Organ transplantation*. Westport, CT: Greenwood Press.

Polit, D.F., & Beck, C.T. (2012) *Nursing research: Generating and assessing evidence for nursing practice* (9th ed.). Philadelphia: Wolters Kluwer, Lippincott Williams & Wilkins.

United Network for Organ Sharing (UNOS). (2009). *Amended and restated articles of incorporation of United Network for Organ Sharing*. Retrieved from http://www.unos.org/docs/UNOS_ArticlesOfIncorporation_062309.pdf

United Network for Organ Sharing (UNOS). *2012 United Network for Organ Sharing: Annual report*. Retrieved from http://www.unos.org/docs/AnnualReport2012.pdf

United Network for Organ Sharing (UNOS). (n.d.-a). *About us*. Retrieved from http://www.unos.org/about/index.php

United Network for Organ Sharing (UNOS). (n.d.-b). *Donation and transplantation*. Retrieved from http://www.unos.org/donation/index.php

United Network for Organ Sharing (UNOS). (n.d.-c). *History*. Retrieved from http://www.unos.org/donation/index.php?topic=history

United Network for Organ Sharing (UNOS). (n.d.-d). *Professional education*. Retrieved from http://www.unos.org/donation/index.php?topic=professional_education

United Network for Organ Sharing (UNOS). (n.d.-e). *Services and capabilities*. Retrieved from http://www.unos.org/services/index.php

United Network for Organ Sharing (UNOS). (n.d.-f). *UNOS facts and figures.* Retrieved from http://www.unos.org/docs/UNOS_FactsFigures.pdf

United States Renal Data System (USRDS). (n.d.-a) *About USRDS.* http://www. usrds.org/About.aspx

United States Renal Data System (USRDS).(n.d.-b). *Frequently asked questions.* http://www.usrds.org/faq.aspx

United States Renal Disease System (USRDS). (2012). *2012 Atlas of CKD and ESRD.* Retrieved from http://www.usrds.org/atlas12.aspx

United States Renal Data System (USRDS). (2013). *2013 annual data report* (Vols. 1 & 2). Retrieved from http://www.usrds.org/adr.aspx

University of Michigan Kidney Epidemiology and Cost Center (UM-KECC). (n.d.) *History of UM-KECC.* Retrieved from http://kecc.sph.umich.edu/about-us/mission

CHAPTER **3**

Health Policy, Politics, and Influence in Nephrology Nursing

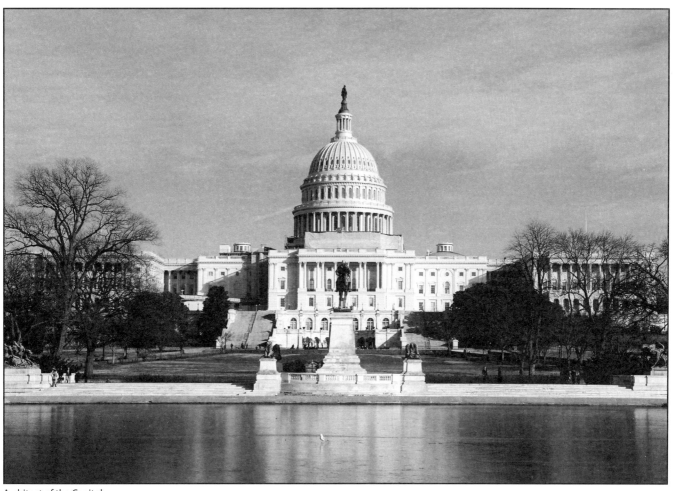

Architect of the Capitol

Chapter Editor and Author

Donna Bednarski, MSN, RN, ANP-BC, CNN, CNP

CHAPTER 3
Health Policy, Politics, and Influence in Nephrology Nursing

This offering for **1.8 contact hours** is provided by the American Nephrology Nurses' Association (ANNA).

American Nephrology Nurses' Association is accredited as a provider of continuing nursing education by the American Nurses Credentialing Center Commission on Accreditation.

ANNA is a provider approved by the California Board of Registered Nursing, provider number CEP 00910.

This CNE offering meets the continuing nursing education requirements for certification and recertification by the Nephrology Nursing Certification Commission (NNCC).

To be awarded contact hours for this activity, read this chapter in its entirety. Then complete the CNE evaluation found at **www.annanurse.org/corecne** and submit it; or print it, complete it, and mail it in. Contact hours are not awarded until the evaluation for the activity is complete.

Example of reference for Chapter 3 in APA format. One author for entire chapter.

Bednarski, D. (2015). Health policy, politics, and influence in nephrology nursing. In C.S. Counts (Ed.), *Core curriculum for nephrology nursing: Module 1: Foundations for practice in nephrology nursing* (6th ed., pp. 87-108). Pitman, NJ: American Nephrology Nurses' Association.

Interpreted: Chapter author. (Date). Title of chapter. In ...

Cover photo: Courtesy of Architect of the Capitol, http://www.aoc.gov/image-gallery

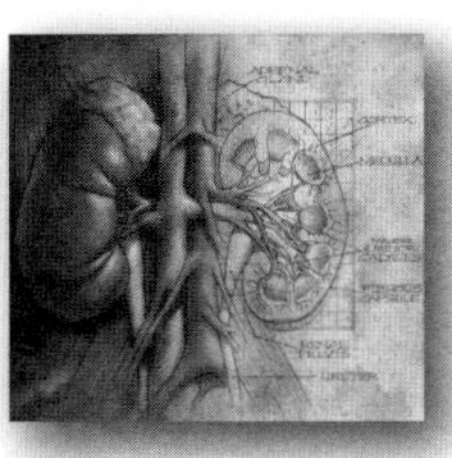

CHAPTER 3
Health Policy, Politics, and Influence in Nephrology Nursing

Purpose

The purpose of this chapter is multifaceted. A primary purpose is to familiarize the reader with the important role played by federal and state governments in providing coverage for the treatment of kidney disease. It is the responsibility of professional nurses to advocate for policies, including reimbursement policies, which support the provision of high quality care. The chapter will also provide an overview of the legislative process, communicating with members of Congress and other policymakers, and ANNA's involvement in health policy. ANNA is a leader in advocacy for nephrology nursing and individuals with kidney disease and their families. By engaging with federal and state legislators, government agencies, and other organizations, nephrology nurses can continue to influence policies critical to nephrology professionals, patients, and their families.

Objectives

Upon completion of this chapter, the learner will be able to:
1. Define basic terms used in the legislative process.
2. Outline the policy and political process.
3. Describe opportunities to be politically active.
4. Describe current factors impacting healthcare policy.

SECTION A
Advocacy

I. Facets of advocacy.

A. *Advocacy* is a term used for organized activism related to a particular set of issues. Advocacy, therefore, supports or defends a cause (ANNA, 2013a).

B. Advocacy requires understanding the issue, identifying goals, and communicating them to others.

C. It is every nurse's professional responsibility to act as a patient advocate (ANA, 2001; Ulrich, 2011). Policy advocacy is an important component of such advocacy.

D. The purpose of being a policy advocate includes:
1. Providing expert representation on an issue.
2. Ensuring that facts are presented in a manner that enables legislators and other policymakers to make informed decisions.
3. Promoting legislation and other policies on the state and federal levels.

II. Importance of involvement.

A. Much of the professional lives of nurses is and will continue to be influenced by legislation and regulation at both the state and national levels.

B. Patient care is a highly political endeavor. It determines who gets care, type of care, and by whom (Mason et al., 2007).

C. Congress makes decisions that affect the health care of the nation, yet few Members of Congress are knowledgeable about health care. Nurses can play key roles in educating and influencing policymakers. Nurses who work in nephrology possess expert knowledge in the care and needs of persons with kidney disease.

D. As the largest group of healthcare providers, nurses have tremendous power to influence legislation and other policy.

E. Gallup's annual poll (2012), reflecting the opinion of the general public, found that nurses top the honesty and ethics list.

F. It is critical that nurses speak up about healthcare issues they face daily, such as quality patient care, patient satisfaction, outcomes of care, adequate staffing, safe workplaces, environments, etc. (Abood, 2007).

G. Nurses can provide valid information on the needs of the healthcare system and methods to improve patient care.

H. As challenging and time-consuming as healthcare policy advocacy can be, the process offers many opportunities for active participation and making an impact that increases control over patient care and outcomes (Abood, 2007).

I. With growing economic constraints, nurses are in a position to advocate for patients in access, quality, or cost (Ulrich, 2011).

III. Arenas of involvement (Mason et al., 2007).

A. Workplace: impacting how care is provided and by whom.
   1. Input into policies and procedures.
   2. Involvement in decision making at all levels of the institution through shared decision-making models.

B. Community: the ability to impact a better place for citizens to live, participating in activities such as:
   1. Parent-teacher associations, community planning boards, involvement in civic organizations, and business groups.
   2. Addressing issues such as recycling, environmental cleanup, and safety.

C. Professional organizations: offer one avenue through which individual nurses and the profession as a whole can work together to achieve power and influence policy. They are instrumental in shaping nursing practice.
   1. Develop standards of practice.
   2. Address broader health and social issues and provide a national presence.
   3. Achieve increased influence with increased nurses' involvement.

D. Government: impacting all areas of care provision on the local, state, and federal levels.
   1. Impacts all aspects of our lives (e.g., mandatory immunizations, and healthcare services eligibility).
   2. Determines the definition of nursing.
   3. Defines who receives care, under what circumstances, and what type of health services they may receive.

Section B
Advocacy History of ANNA

I. 1980s.

A. ANNA was known as the American Association of Nephrology Nurses and Technicians (AANNT).

B. The first position statements were published in 1983. Position statements represent succinct summaries of the organization's stand on an issue for the purpose of influence, advocacy, and/or clarification. The first position statements supported:
   1. The use of advanced practice nurses.
   2. Cost-containment efforts.
   3. Efforts to increase organ donation.

C. Initiation of the Legislative Committee, 1987.

D. Establishment of the Legislative Consultant role, 1988.

II. 1990s.

A. The initiation of ANNA legislative workshops, which were held every other year.

B. The first legislative handbook was published.

C. The Legislative Representative was added to the roster of chapter officers.

D. The State Director role was instituted.

E. The legislative advisors were added to the roster of regional officers.

F. Development of the ANNA Health Policy Statement and Health Policy Agenda. Both documents are reviewed and updated annually and can be found on the ANNA website.

III. 2000s.

A. Establishment of the state legislative consultant, 2000.

B. In 2003, ANNA purchased and began maintaining CapWiz, which can be found on the ANNA website. ANNA maintains the CapWiz Legislative Action Center so members can communicate quickly and easily with their elected representatives about issues that have an impact on individuals with kidney disease and nephrology nursing practice.

C. Education for state and federal lawmakers. The first End Stage Renal Disease (ESRD) Education Day was held in August 2003.
   1. This initiative was dedicated to educating legislators and other policymakers about kidney disease, treatment options, and legislative issues facing the kidney community. Members are encouraged to invite Congressional delegations, Centers for Medicare and Medicaid Services (CMS) staff, ESRD regional office staff, local elected officials, and regulatory agency staff to visit a local dialysis facility and/or transplant center.
   2. The day allows all willing nephrology nurses, from bedside to administration, to share their knowledge of patient care and participate in policy advocacy.
   3. Since the initial ESRD Education Day, hundreds of federal, state, and city officials and their staffs have toured dialysis facilities nationwide.
   4. ESRD Education Day grew to ESRD Education Week by August 2005, with other organizations and associations participating in the educational endeavor.
   5. Name changed to Kidney Disease Awareness and Education Week in 2008. The focus continues to be dedicated to educating policymakers and their staff members about the needs of patients suffering from, or at risk for, ESRD.

D. Terminology changes, 2004.
   1. ANNA Legislative Committee became the Health Policy Committee.
   2. Legislative Consultant became Health Policy Consultant.
   3. State Legislative Consultant became State Health Policy Consultant.
   4. Legislative Advisors became Health Policy Advisors.
   5. State Directors became Health Policy State Directors.
   6. Legislative Representatives became Health Policy Representatives.

E. Updates to Health Policy Committee. The addition of the following volunteer roles:
   1. Advisor for Position Statements.
   2. Advisor for Kidney Disease Awareness and Education Week.
   3. Advisor for CapWiz.

F. The initiation of the ANNA Capitol Gang. The ANNA Capitol Gang is a group of ANNA volunteer nurses who have experience speaking with legislators and the ability to get to Washington, DC, at a "moment's notice" to discuss issues on behalf of ANNA.

G. Development of the ANNA Resource Corps (ARC) designed to match the unique talents and skills of its volunteer members with volunteer opportunities for the association.

H. Increased ANNA health policy activities. Refer to ANNA website: http://www.annanurse.org. For a list of recent activities, choose Advocacy, then Endorsements or Legislative Priorities. Sample activities include:
   1. Contribution by ANNA to regulatory language with formation of task forces to review legislative documents.
   2. Comment on federal legislative initiatives.
      a. Kidney Care Quality and Improvement Act of 2005.
      b. The Kidney Care Quality and Education Act of 2007.
      c. Join the nursing community on issues:
         (1) Nursing education, such as the appropriation of funds for the Nurse Reinvestment Act.
         (2) Funding for Title VIII programs, nursing workforce development programs.
      d. Support Kidney Care Partners on issues.
      e. Centers for Medicare & Medicaid Services (CMS) annual proposed rules to Medicare Program; End-Stage Renal Disease (ESRD) Quality Incentive Program (QIP) and End-Stage Renal Disease Prospective Payment System (ESRD PPS).
   3. Support for state legislative initiatives.
      a. Letter sent to the National Council of State Boards of Nursing in support of State Licensure Compacts.
      b. Response letters to the role of unlicensed personnel in dialysis.
   4. Input into regulatory agencies' activities (e.g., response to the Joint Commission Field Review: Organ Transplant Center Certification, 2006).
   5. Endorsements of nursing organization standards (e.g., endorsement of AACN Standards for Establishing and Sustaining Healthy Work Environments, 2006).

6. Member of Kidney Care Partners (KCP).
   a. Founded in May of 2003 and located in Washington, DC, KCP is a coalition of patient advocates, dialysis professionals, providers, and suppliers working together to improve the quality of care for individuals with chronic kidney disease (CKD).
   b. KCP mission, individually and collectively, is to ensure:
      (1) Patients with CKD receive optimal care.
      (2) Patients with CKD are able to live quality lives.
      (3) Dialysis care is readily accessible to all those in need.
      (4) Research and development leads to enhanced therapies and innovative products.
   c. Partners include organizations from the nephrology community.
      (1) Patient advocacy organizations (e.g., National Kidney Foundation, American Kidney Fund, Renal Support Network, Dialysis Patient Citizens).
      (2) Professional organizations (e.g., ANNA, Renal Physicians Association, American Society of Nephrology, American Society of Pediatric Nephrology).
      (3) Dialysis suppliers (e.g., DaVita HealthPartners Inc., Fresenius Medical Care North America, Northwest Kidney Centers, Dialysis Clinic, Inc.).
      (4) Manufacturers (e.g., Amgen, Genzyme).
   d. More information can be found on the KCP website: http://www.kidneycarepartners.org

I. Second week of September established as Nephrology Nurses Week.
   1. Initiated in 2005 to honor the dedicated nephrology nurses who care for patients with kidney disease.
   2. ANNA launched Nephrology Nurses Week to give employers, patients, and others the opportunity to thank nephrology nurses for their life-saving work.
   3. Celebrates the many skills of the nephrology nurse at the bedside and in patient advocacy.
   4. Sample activities.
      a. ANNA chapter-sponsored educational sessions.
      b. Structured recognitions and awards.
      c. Distribution of Nephrology Nurses Week products or other ANNA items.
      d. Thank-you notes to nephrology nurses.
      e. Games and prizes.
      f. Ice cream socials.
   5. Additional resources can be found on the ANNA website, including:
      a. Nephrology Nurses Week online toolkit.
         (1) Nephrology Nurses Week logo.
         (2) Nephrology Nurses Week poster.
         (3) Nephrology Nurses Week press release.
         (4) Nephrology Nurses Week newsletter article.
         (5) Nephrology Nurses Week proclamation.
         (6) Nephrology Nurses Week Letter to Local Media (print, television, or radio).
      b. Nephrology Nurses Week products.
      c. How You Celebrate Nephrology Nurses Week survey to share experiences.

J. In December 2005, the firm of Gardner, Carton & Douglas was retained as the legislative consulting firm for ANNA. The firm's name changed in 2007 to Drinker Biddle & Reath LLP. Activities of firm:
   1. Helps increase ANNA member involvement, understanding, and appreciation by explaining the issues and the need to engage in advocacy at the grassroots level.
   2. Engages in activities on ANNA's behalf.
   3. Monitors legislative and regulatory activities that are perceived to have a direct impact on the practice of nephrology nursing and the ESRD program, CKD, transplantation, and related therapies.
   4. Reviews, analyzes, and evaluates proposed legislation that affects ANNA and its interests and make recommendations regarding courses of action.
   5. Represents ANNA before Congress, federal agencies, and the nursing and nephrology communities.
   6. Assists in the development of position statements and revision of ANNA's legislative platform.
   7. Serves as a member of the Health Policy Committee.

IV. 2010s.

A. Changes in ANNA.
   1. In 2012, members approved the reorganization of the ANNA governance structure, with elimination of regions to allow all members to vote for all Board members.
   2. Development of Specialty Practice Networks (SPNs): provide members opportunities to network with other members in various nephrology subspecialties. Provides an opportunity for discussing nursing issues/concerns and collaborate to create solutions to current practice challenges.
   3. Elimination of roles: Capitol Gang, State Health Policy Consultant, State Director.

B. Joined as a pioneer member of the Kidney Health Initiative. In 2012, organized by the American

Society of Nephrology to advance scientific understanding of kidney health and patient safety implications of new and innovative drugs, devices, and treatments by creating a collaborative environment with the FDA and the greater nephrology community.

C. Forged new connections with the Centers for Medicare & Medicaid Services and the Center for Medicare & Medicaid Innovation.

D. Joined as member of National Quality Forum, 2013.

E. Hosted first Virtual Lobby Day, 2013.

F. The Health Policy Committee composition changed in 2013 to the following:
   1. Chairperson, Chairperson Designate, Federal Health Policy Consultant, and six Health Policy Advisors.
   2. Committee coordinates the annual Kidney Disease Awareness Education week.
   3. Committee coordinates the Position Statement development and revisions.

G. Continued ANNA health policy activities. Refer to ANNA website: http://www.annanurse.org. For a list of recent activities, choose Advocacy, then Endorsements or Legislative Priorities. Sample activities include:
   1. Support for federal legislative initiatives.
   2. Support for state legislative initiatives.
   3. Input into regulatory agencies' activities.
   4. Continued collaboration with the nursing community.
   5. Collaboration with nephrology community organizations.
   6. Continued activity and member of Kidney Care Partners (KCP).
   7. Continued relationship with Drinker Biddle & Reath LLP; additional role includes:
      a. Participates in and represents ANNA before Kidney Care Partners, the nursing community, and other various coalitions as requested.
      b. Analyzes proposed federal regulations and assists ANNA in drafting written comments to the appropriate agency.
      c. Leads the efforts to plan and implement of the biannual ANNA Health Policy Workshop.
      d. Attends and presents on health policy issues at the annual National Symposium.
      e. Drafts a quarterly health policy article for publication.

Section C
Public Policy and the Political Process

Part 1. "Civics 101"

I. Basic terminology.

A. Constituent – an individual who appoints or elects another as their representative or agent.

B. Bill – legislation introduced in either federal or state legislatures.

C. Authorization bill – legislation that formally establishes a program or activity and obligates funding for such. An authorization may be effective for 1 year, a fixed number of years, or an indefinite period. An authorization may be for a specified amount of funds or for "such sums as may be necessary."

D. Appropriations bill – legislation that formally approves the provision of funds from the United States Treasury for an authorized program or activity.

E. Sponsor – the original legislator who introduced a bill.

F. Cosponsor – a legislator (or legislators) who formally add his/her name in support of another legislator's bill.

G. Amendment – to change a bill by adding, deleting, or substituting portions of it.

H. Committee – a group of legislators assigned to review certain bills.

I. Act – legislation that has been passed into law.

J. Veto – power to say no or forbid.

II. Characteristics of U.S. Congress.

Bicameral – consists of two chambers, the Senate and the House of Representatives. All states with the exception of Nebraska are also bicameral. See Table 3.1.

III. Enacting legislation.

A. There are three branches of government.
   1. The executive branch includes the president, vice president, federal departments, and agencies.
   2. The judicial branch is a court system for the interpretation of laws.
   3. The legislative branch is Congress with the primary purpose to make laws.

Table 3.1

Bicameral Legislative System

	U.S. House of Representatives	U.S. Senate
Referred to as	1. Representative. 2. Congressman or Congresswoman.	1. Senator. 2. Member of Congress.
Numbers	1. 435 individuals determined by the Federal Census and reviewed every 10 years. 2. The District of Columbia and U.S. territories (Guam, Puerto Rico, Samoa, Virgin Islands) each have a single delegate. 3. All states have at least one representative.	1. 100 individuals, 2 from each state. 2. No senator from U.S. territories or the District of Columbia.
Term	1. 2 years. 2. All members elected every 2 years.	1. 6 years. 2. One third elected every 2 years.
Eligibility	1. Age 25 or older. 2. U.S. citizen for 7 years. 3. Resides in the district representing.	1. Age 30 or older. 2. U.S. citizen for 9 years. 3. Resides in the district representing.

Source: United States House of Representatives: http://www.house.gov United States Senate: http://www.senate.gov

B. Introducing legislation.
   1. There are two main types of legislation: authorizing bill and appropriations bill.
      a. How a bill becomes law (refer below) generally applies to both authorizing and appropriations legislation.
      b. For a law to be enacted, it must be passed by both chambers and signed by the president.
      c. Before money can be spent, Congress must authorize the expenditure and then appropriate the funds to do so. This formal process consists of two sequential steps.
         (1) Enactment of authorization of a program or activity. Legislative committees from both chambers are responsible for authorizing legislation related to agencies and programs under their jurisdiction.
         (2) Enactment of appropriations to provide funds for the authorized program or activity. The Appropriations committees of the House and Senate have jurisdiction over appropriations measures.
   2. Bills are drafts of proposed legislation that are introduced in either the House or Senate (Smith, 2006).
      a. They create public policies.
      b. Ideas can come from any citizen.
      c. Can be introduced by any member of Congress.
      d. Bills introduced in the House are labeled with "HR" and followed by a number.
      e. Bills introduced in the Senate are labeled with an "S" and followed by a number.
      f. While thousands of bills are introduced into congressional session, very few are enacted into law.
      g. If a bill is not acted upon over the course of the 2-year session of Congress, it "dies" at the end of the session and must be reintroduced in the next session.

C. How a bill becomes law (ANNA, 2013a).
   1. After being introduced, bills are assigned a number and labeled with a sponsor's name. The bill may have a cosponsor or cosponsors, but they are not required.
   2. The Speaker of the House or the Presiding Officer

in the Senate will then assign the bill to the committee with jurisdiction over the subject.
   a. Bills may be referred to more than one committee and may be split so that parts are sent to different committees and subsequently to subcommittees.
   b. The major work of reviewing and modifying bills is done in committee.
   c. If there is failure of the committee to act on a bill, the bill will "die in committee." This happens frequently if grassroots and member support is not highly visible.
3. Activities within the committee.
   a. Subcommittee hearings and markups.
      (1) Hearings. Subcommittees have the option to hold hearings on a bill and invite testimony from public and private witnesses.
      (2) Markups. Once hearings are complete, subcommittee members go through the measure line-by-line, marking up adopted changes.
      (3) Subcommittee members vote on whether to report the bill favorably to the full committee. If the vote is not favorably reported, the bill usually dies.
   b. Full committee hearings and markups.
      (1) The full committee may repeat any or all of the subcommittee's procedures: hearings, markups, and a vote.
      (2) If there are substantial revisions, the committee can introduce a "clean bill." The new bill will be assigned a new number.
      (3) If the full committee votes favorably, it is reported to the whole chamber, House, or Senate.
4. Floor action.
   a. The bill is brought to the Senate or House floor for debate.
      (1) The bill may be amended.
      (2) Voted up or down.
      (3) Referred back to committee or tabled. If these options occur, the bill usually dies.
   b. The bill is then voted on and passed by majority vote. It is sent to the other chamber unless the other chamber already has a similar bill under consideration. If it fails, then the bill usually dies.
   c. If both chambers, the House and Senate, pass the same bill, then it is sent to the president. However, if the bills are not the same and they both pass, they are sent to a conference committee to work out the differences between the two bills. Most major legislation goes to a conference committee (Kuchta et al., 2006).
      (1) The bills move to conference committee for further review and amending.
      (2) The conference committee is made up of members from each chamber.
      (3) If the conference committee is unable to reach an agreement with changes or amendments, the bill usually dies.
      (4) If the conference committee reaches a compromise, it completes a conference report, which is sent back to each chamber. Both the House and the Senate must approve the conference report or the bill usually dies.
   d. After the bill has been approved by both the House and Senate, it is sent to the president.
5. Presidential and congressional actions (Kuchta et al., 2006).
   a. The president can sign the bill into law.
   b. If the president takes no action within 10 days while Congress is in session, the bill dies.
   c. If the president takes no action within 10 days after Congress has adjourned, the bill does not become law. This is called a "pocket veto."
   d. The president can veto the bill and send it back to Congress with recommendations.
   e. Congress can override a veto with two-thirds vote.

D. After a law is passed.
1. It is referred to the appropriate executive branch agency for the development of regulations for the purpose of implementing the law.
   a. Agencies prepare proposed rules in advance of regulatory action.
   b. The draft is circulated for review.
   c. Once cleared, the proposed rule is printed in the Federal Register, a document used to notify the public of all proposed rules, administrative matters, and selected presidential activities. The Federal Register lists:
      (1) The regulating agency.
      (2) The name of the proposed rule.
      (3) The summary of the regulatory action.
      (4) Any needed background information.
      (5) A contact person at the agency.
   d. The public usually has 30 to 60 days to respond to a proposed rule, allowing another opportunity for grassroots/member involvement.
   e. Each of the comments is reviewed, and a final rule is developed.
   f. The final rule is published in the Federal Registry, specifying an effective date for implementation. A summary of public comments to the proposed rule is included. Table 3.2 delineates events in legislative history and regulatory history that have impacted the patient with kidney disease.

Table 3.2

Events in Legislative History That Have Impacted the Kidney Patient (page 1 of 4)

Title of Legislation	Important Dates	Key Points
Gottschalk Committee	1967	■ Responsible for considering all aspects of the problems posed by CKD and making recommendations toward managing them. ■ Recommendations. 1. Initiate a national program for the treatment of ESRD. 2. Finance the program by amending the Social Security Act to "cover the permanently disabled regardless of age." 3. Deem persons with CKD as disabled, thereby entitling patients with ESRD to Medicare benefits.
HR-1: Social Security Amendments of 1972	1. ESRD amendment introduced September 30, 1972. 2. House-Senate conference report issued October 14, 1972. 3. HR-1 became Public Law 92-603 when signed by President Nixon on October 30, 1972. 4. Effective date for Medicare coverage for chronic kidney failure was July 1, 1973.	■ Intent of Medicare coverage. 1. Provide equitable access for all patients with ESRD. 2. Patients who were certified to have chronic kidney failure and require dialysis or transplantation by a physician were deemed disabled. 3. Entitled to Medicare Part A and Part B benefits via Medicare disability program. 4. Premium paid by beneficiary for Part B benefits.
Conditions of participation	Interim regulations: June 29, 1973	1. Interim conditions of participation and payment rates for dialysis and transplant services.
	Interim regulations: April 22, 1975	1. Minor modifications to and republication of initial interim regulations concerning coverage of services.
	NPRM: July 1, 1975	1. Specified conditions of coverage that facilities must meet to qualify for Medicare reimbursement. 2. Included health and safety requirements. 3. Directed the organization of the ESRD Network System.
	Final rule: June 3, 1976	1. Finalized condition of participation as ESRD provider/supplies and coverage.
	Final rule: August 11, 1978	1. Authorized temporary approval as kidney transplantation centers for pediatric hospitals. 2. Allowed for Medicare approval/reimbursement without meeting the required minimal utilization for number of kidney transplants performed.
Social Security Act Amendment	1978	1. Department of Health, Education and Welfare directed to establish: a. Incentive based or prospective dialysis systems. b. Payments required to be on a cost related or economical and equitable basis. 2. Extended Medicare transplant benefits from 12 to 36 months posttransplant.
Omnibus Budget Reconciliation Act	1981	1. Established composite rate effective 8/1/1983. A single rate to cover all supplies and services. This included home and in-center dialysis treatments. 2. Payment averaged $127 per treatment ($11 per treatment reduction).

Table continues

Table 3.2

Events in Legislative History That Have Impacted the Kidney Patient (page 2 of 4)

Title of Legislation	Important Dates	Key Points
Prospective composite rate payment system	NPRM: February 12, 1982 Final rule: May 11, 1983	1. Established a payment rate per treatment adjusted for geographic wage differences. 2. Separate rates for hospital-based and independent dialysis facilities. 3. Exception process developed based on atypical patient mix, extraordinary circumstances, education costs, or as an isolated essential facility. 4. Physician payment modified to a single monthly prospective capitation payment (MCP).
National Organ Transplant Act of 1984	1984	■ Public Law 98-507. 1. Created task force on organ transplantation. 2. Amended the Public Health Service Act to authorize the Secretary of Health and Human Services (HHS) to make grants for the establishment, initial operation, and expansion planning of qualified organ procurement organizations (OPOs). 3. Directed the Secretary of the HHS to: a. Establish an Organ Procurement and Transplantation Network (OPTN) to provide a central registry linking donors and potential recipients. b. Establish a scientific registry of organ recipients. c. Designate and maintain an identifiable unit in the Public Health service to coordinate federal organ transplant programs and policies. d. Publish an annual report on the scientific and clinical status of organ transplantation. 4. Prohibited the purchase or sale of human organs if such transfer affects interstate commerce and established criminal penalties for such violations.
Omnibus Budget Reconciliation Act (OBRA) of 1986 (ESRD provisions)	1986	■ Legislated via Public Law 99-609. 1. Amended section 1881 of the Social Security Act. 2. Authorized Secretary of HHS to set composite rate for dialysis services provided between October 1, 1986, and October 1, 1988, at a level equal to the rate in effect as of May 13, 1986, reduced by $2. 3. Reduced the composite payment rate by an additional $0.50 to finance the Network administrative organization. 4. Required a study to evaluate the effects of the payment reductions on access and quality of care (due January 1, 1988). 5. Established a national ESRD registry to assemble and analyze data, known as U.S. Renal Data System (USRDS). 6. Modified/reorganized the Network Administration Organization. 7. Extended coverage of immunosuppressive drugs. 8. Established protocols or standards and conditions for safe and effective dialyzer reuse. 9. Established organ procurement protocols as a requirement for hospitals and organizations involved in procuring organs for transplantations.
Omnibus Budget Reconciliation Act	1986	1. Reduced payment $2 per treatment for 2 years (1987 and 1988). 2. Reimbursement reduced $.50 per treatment to fund ESRD Networks permanently.
Final rule: ESRD Networks	August 26, 1986	1. Authorized the Secretary of HHS to designate the ESRD Network areas. 2. Delineated 14 network areas and criteria used to determine these areas. 3. OBRA of 1986 required modification to at least 17 Network organizations.

Table continues

Table 3.2

Events in Legislative History That Have Impacted the Kidney Patient (page 3 of 4)

Title of Regulation	Important Dates	Key Points
Final rule: Reuse	October 1, 1987	1. Standards for the reuse of hemodialyzers, filters, and other dialysis supplies.
Notice for Proposed Rule Making (NPRM): Occupational exposure to bloodborne pathogens	May 30, 1989	1. Infection control plan must be designed and implemented by each employer to minimize or eliminate employee exposure. 2. Plan shall be reviewed and updated as needed. 3. Universal precautions shall be observed inclusive of: a. Hand washing as frequently as needed. b. Use of personal protective equipment. • Gloves. • Masks, eye protection, and face shields.
Omnibus Budget Reconciliation Act	1989	1. Maintained the $2 treatment reduction through 1990. 2. Gramm Rudman Hollings 2% sequestration also began in 1989.
Budget Law	1990	1. Continued sequester through December 31, 1990. 2. Increased rate $1 per treatment for 1991. 3. Established a statutory payment rate for EPO at $11 per thousand units.
Omnibus Budget Reconciliation Act	1993	Reduced the statutory payment rate for EPO to $10 per thousand units.
Balanced Budget Refinement Act	1999	Increased rate 2.4% over 2 years (2000 and 2001).
Beneficiary Improvement and Protection Act	2000	1. Increased rate additional 1.2% for 2001. 2. Directed the development of a market basket. 3. Directed HHS to develop a system to bundle some separately payable drugs into the composite rate.
Medicare Modernization Act (MMA)	2003	1. 1.5% increase for 2005. 2. Beginning in 2005, required "drug add-on" to composite rate, basing payment on the Average Sales Price plus 6%. 3. Called for a fully bundled dialysis prospective payment system (PPS), incorporating all separately billable items and services into the dialysis payment.
Deficit Reduction Act	2005	1. 1.6% increase for 2006. 2. Drug add-on increased 1.4% in 2006.
Medicare Program; Conditions for Coverage for End Stage Renal Disease (ESRD) Facilities; Proposed Rule; CMS-3818-P	NPRM: February 4, 2005	1. This proposed rule would revise the requirements that ESRD dialysis facilities must meet to be certified under the Medicare program. 2. The revised requirements focus on the patient, including: a. The results of the care provided to the patient. b. Establish performance expectations for facilities. c. Encourage patients to participate in their care plan and treatment. d. Eliminate many procedural requirements from the current conditions for coverage. e. Preserve strong process measures when necessary to promote patient well being and continuous quality improvement. 3. Changes are necessary to reflect the advances in dialysis technology and standard care practices since the requirements were last revised in their entirety in 1976.

Table continues

Table 3.2

Events in Legislative History That Have Impacted the Kidney Patient (page 4 of 4)

Title of Regulation	Important Dates	Key Points
Medicare Program; Hospital Conditions of Participation: Requirements for Approval and Re-approval of Transplant Centers to Perform Organ Transplants; Proposed Rule; CMS-3835-P	NPRM: February 4, 2005 Final: March 30, 2007 Effective: June 28, 2007	1. Establishes, for the first time, Medicare conditions of participation for heart, heart–lung, intestine, kidney, liver, lung, and pancreas transplant centers. 2. Sets forth clear expectations for minimal health and safety rules to provide safe, high quality transplant service delivery in all Medicare-participating facilities.
Proposed Rule for Revisions to Payment Policies Under the Physician Fee Schedule for Calendar Year (CY) 2006	Federal Register: September 1, 2005	This document corrects errors in the proposed rule that appeared in the Federal Register on August 8, 2005, entitled "Medicare Program; Revisions to Payment Policies Under the Physician Fee Schedule for Calendar Year 2006."
Tax Relief and Health Care Act	2006	1. 1.6% increase beginning April 2007. 2. Drug add-on increased 0.5% in 2007.
Medicare Improvements for Patients and Providers Act (MIPPA)	2008	1. Required Medicare to establish a full PPS for ESRD services to include composite rate components, injectable drugs and biologics and their oral equivalents, laboratory tests, and renal-related oral medications. 2. Created the ESRD PPS to be effective 1/1/2011, reducing payment by 2% with base rate $229.63 before wage adjustment. 3. Drug add-on increased 0.5%. 4. Increased composite rate 1% for 2009 and an additional 1% in 2010. 5. Created an annual market basket update to the PPS payment rate minus 1% beginning 2012 (Accountable Care Act 2010 reduced the update by a productivity adjustment factor). 6. Established the Quality Incentive Program (QIP); ESRD providers to meet certain quality metrics, to be defined annually, effective in 2012. Facilities failing to meet defined metrics may lose up to 2% for total Medicare reimbursement for a payment year.
The American Taxpayer Relief Act (ATRA)	2012	1. Medicare is required to recalculate the dialysis bundled payment rate for 2014 to account for changes in drug and biological use as a result of the PPS. 2. Delayed inclusion of oral drugs into the ESRD PPS.

Source: ANNA, 2013c; Swaminathan et al., 2012
Bundling: http://cms.hhs.gov/Medicare/Medicare-Fee-for-Service-Payment/ESRDpayment/index.html

IV. Federal budget.

A. Budgets are prepared by each federal agency and submitted to the Office of Management and Budget (OMB). OMB then finalizes the proposed funding levels based on the priorities of the president.
   1. Three main components.
      a. How much the federal government should spend on public purposes.
      b. How much it should take in as tax revenue.
      c. Identification of the deficit or surplus the federal government should run.
   2. The president's budget spells out how much funding is recommended for each "discretionary" or "appropriated" program.
      a. These programs fall under the jurisdiction of the House and Senate Appropriations committees.
      b. To continue operating, any discretionary program must have funding renewed each year or at the previously defined interval.
      c. Discretionary programs make up about one third of all federal spending and include programs such as defense spending, health research, and housing.
   3. The president's budget can also include changes to "mandatory" or "entitlement" programs (e.g., Social Security, Medicare, Medicaid, food stamps, military retirement benefits, unemployment insurance). Entitlement programs are not controlled by annual appropriations.
   4. The president's budget can also include changes to the tax code. Any proposal to increase or decrease taxes should be reflected in the change in federal revenue over the following and future years.

B. In early February, the president submits this budget to the House and the Senate budget committees (Smith, 2006).
   1. The House and Senate Budget committees are to draft the budget resolution.
   2. Once completed, the resolution goes to the House and Senate where it can be amended.
   3. Once both houses pass the resolution, it goes to the House-Senate conference to reconcile any differences, and a conference report is developed.
   4. Once approved, it does not go to the president for signature or veto. It requires only a majority vote to pass. As a result, no funds are appropriated. The budget resolution serves as a template for the actual appropriation process.
   5. The budget resolution is to be passed by April 15, but it often takes longer. The federal fiscal year begins on October 1.
   6. If Congress does not pass a budget resolution, a "continuing resolution" is usually passed. The continuing resolution temporarily funds federal programs at some agreed upon rate or previous year's level, until the appropriations bills are passed.
   7. The budget committees are required by law to issue two budget resolutions each year.
      a. The initial resolution defines revenue and spending.
      b. Later in the year, this resolution is updated to reflect actual economic data.

C. If government spending exceeds the parameters of the budget resolution, budget reconciliation is needed to balance the budget.
   1. Historically, health programs are dramatically affected by this activity.
   2. Each authorizing committee targets specific areas of "savings." Often program changes are voted on as well as legislation passed to authorize spending.

D. Budget reconciliation.
   1. An optional process that Congress may use to assure compliance with direct spending, revenue, and debt limit levels set forth in the budget resolution.
   2. If Congress decides to use the reconciliation process, language known as a "reconciliation directive" must be included in the budget resolution. The reconciliation directive instructs various committees to produce legislation by a specified date to achieve the goals in budget resolution.

V. Other resources.

http://www.annanurse.org
http://www.firstgov.org
http://www.congress.org
http://thomas.loc.gov
http://vote-smart.org/index.htm

Part 2. State Government

I. Powers under the state government.

A. States must take responsibility for:
   1. Ownership of property.
   2. Education of inhabitants.
   3. Implementation of welfare and other benefits programs and distribution of aid.
   4. Protection of people from local threats.
   5. Maintenance of a justice system.
   6. Establishment of local governments (counties and municipalities).
   7. Maintenance of state highways and establishment of a means for administration of local roads.

8. Regulation of industry.
9. Procurement of funds to support these required activities.
10. Administration of mandates set forth by the federal government.

B. Each state must have its own constitution to use as the basis for laws with a means for amending.

II. State variations.

A. Each state has variations in the operation of its government.

B. Legislative salaries range from nothing to large salaries.

C. Health policy sessions also vary among states, ranging from very short sessions (45 days) to longer sessions (6 to 12 months) (ANNA, 2012).

D. There are other elected positions that may include the following.
   1. Lieutenant governor.
   2. Secretary of state.
   3. Attorney general.
   4. Auditor.
   5. Treasurer.
   6. Superintendent of public instruction.

E. State similarities.
   1. Each state has a governor, lieutenant governor, and other appointed or elected officials.
   2. All states except Nebraska are composed of two chambers – a Senate and General Assembly or House of Representatives.
      a. Nebraska is the only state with a unicameral legislature, having only one chamber, the House, and is nonpartisan.
      b. Nonpartisan refers to government officials who do not identify a formal party affiliation or formal alignment with a political party.
   3. Leaders of each house are responsible for referring bills to committee, recognizing speakers in debate, and presiding over deliberations.

F. Nurse practice acts (NPAs).
   1. Nursing practice is governed by the states. Agencies that do so vary from state to state.
   2. NPAs are the most important legal documents for the nursing profession and the individual nurse. NPAs are created with the purpose of protecting the public.
   3. NPAs define what the functions of nursing shall be and set standards for licensure.
   4. Each state has a local board authorized to formulate and enforce the rules and regulations governing the nursing profession.

G. Nurse Licensure Compact (NLC) (National Council of State Boards of Nursing, 2013).
   1. The Nurse Licensure Compact is a mutual recognition model of nurse licensure allowing a nurse to have one license (in their state of residency) and to practice in multiple states, unless otherwise restricted.
   2. The nurse is subject to each state's practice laws and regulations.
   3. To achieve mutual recognition, each state must enact legislation authorizing the Nurse Licensure Compact.
   4. States entering the compact must also adopt administrative rules and regulations for implementation of the compact.
   5. More information, including participating states, can be found on the National Council of State Boards of Nursing website: https://www.ncsbn.org/index.htm

Part 3. How to Be Politically Active

I. Register and vote in elections.

A. Primary elections are held prior to the general elections and enable voters to select the candidates who will run on each party's ticket.

B. General elections are held to fill public offices.

II. Keep your eyes and ears open. Learn more about state and federal issues that affect your practice and daily life.

A. Sign up for your representative newsletters/mailings/email alerts.

B. Participate in local meet and greets or town hall meetings.

C. Understand the federal and state legislative process. This is the first step in influencing meaningful change (Abood, 2007; Mason et al., 2007).

D. State level.
   1. State board of nursing: Their role is to carry out the nurse practice act to ensure public protection. These activities include determining eligibility for licensure, issuing licenses, approving nurse education programs, investigating complaints, taking disciplinary actions, and determining the scope of practice and licensure for advanced practice registered nurses (APRNs) (Mason et al., 2007).
      a. Contact and offer your assistance.
      b. Obtain a copy of your nurse practice act

through your state board of nursing. A copy can be found on http://www.ncsbn.org (ANNA, 2012).
   (1) Read it. Review the rules on delegation to unlicensed personnel; note that some states have specific delegation rules for dialysis technicians.
   (2) Learn how to advise your state board of nursing regarding changes needed to improve nephrology nursing.
2. State nurses' association (ANNA, 2012).
   a. Review their website and look for resources on state legislature, including:
      (1) Annual state legislative days.
      (2) Internships or fellowships.
   b. Contact them:
      (1) Inform them that ANNA monitors legislation pertinent to ESRD/nursing issues.
      (2) Offer your assistance.
      (3) Ask to be put on their health policy listserv and/or alert list.
   c. Become a member of your state association, which offers additional resources.
3. The State Department is responsible for health oversight (e.g., Department of Public Health, Department of Health Services, Department of Community Health) (ANNA, 2012).
   a. Contact them:
      (1) Ask if there is a Chronic Kidney Disease Advisory Committee.
      (2) Ask for contacts in the department who are responsible for ESRD, including those involved with Certificate of Need.
   b. Offer your assistance to them.
4. Check your state legislative website often to keep in touch with issues pending in the state legislature.
5. Get to know your representatives. Invite them to participate in Kidney Disease Awareness and Education Week. Refer to ANNA website for additional information: http://www.annanurse.org/events/kidney-disease-awareness-and-education-week

E. Federal level.
   1. Get to know your representatives.
   2. Invite them to participate in Kidney Disease Awareness and Education Week.

III. Take advantage of the CapWiz Legislation Center to identify issues important to nephrology nurses. CapWiz Legislation Center can be found on the ANNA website.

A. Email elected officials, including the president and members of Congress.
   1. Type in your ZIP code (helps to identify your representatives) or search by last name.
   2. Create a message to send to the representatives.
   3. There are optional prewritten email templates that ANNA develops on various issues of importance to nephrology nurses or a person with kidney disease. It is best to personalize such email templates.

B. Identify issues and legislation. ANNA scans legislation and provides a listing of the key legislation and initiatives underway that impact your day-to-day practice in nephrology nursing.
   1. Legislative alerts and updates – news and information about important issues.
      a. Personalize email templates developed by ANNA.
      b. Click on the topic of interest and complete the required information. The prewritten template will be sent to the representatives.
   2. Current legislation – summaries and status information about key bills.
   3. Key votes – key Congressional roll call votes.
   4. Capitol Hill basics – tips about communicating with members as well as general information about Hill staffers, the legislative process, and more.

C. Elections and candidates. To find election results, enter your ZIP code or search by state.

D. Media guide.
   1. Find and contact national and local media.
   2. This can be done by using a member's ZIP code, individual search, by entering the name of editors, reporters, or producers, or by organization search by entering the organization name (e.g., newspaper, TV, or radio).

IV. Use ANNA Resources available on the ANNA website, www.annanurse.org

A. Health Policy Agenda: identifies ANNA's priorities for Medicare End-Stage Renal Disease (ESRD) Related Issues and Nursing and General Health Care Issues.

B. Health Policy Statement: represents ANNA's viewpoint on major public policy issues relevant to the treatment of individuals with kidney disease and the practice of professional nephrology nursing. It provides ANNA direction on legislative and regulatory issues on local, state, and national levels.

C. ANNA Position Statements: identify ANNA's position on topics related to general nursing, nephrology nursing, and reimbursement.

D. State Fact Sheets: developed for each state with data on kidney disease incidence for that state. This is one way to educate elected officials to show them information about kidney disease and treatment of kidney failure in their jurisdictions (ANNA, 2012).

E. ANNA Health Policy Toolkit: created to educate, inform, and encourage people interested in healthcare issues to become knowledgeable about the legislative process and become involved in health policy advocacy.

V. Participate in Kidney Disease Awareness and Education Week.

Tools are available to assist in this educational week and can be found on the ANNA website, http://www.annanurse.org

A. *Planning and Orientation Guide* (ANNA, 2013b). A step-by-step guide to assist with all the activities associated with setting up a tour, including instructions for sending tour invitations, how to schedule a tour, how to conduct a tour with a Congressional member, and how to follow up the tour to ensure long-term success.

B. *ESRD Briefing Book for State and Federal Policymakers* (ANNA, 2013b). A guide to kidney disease awareness and education. The booklet presents in lay terms the basics of ESRD and includes information on underlying conditions such as diabetes and hypertension, incidence, and treatment costs.

C. Soliciting for a proclamation.
   1. Tips for getting an official proclamation from your community or state can be found on the ANNA website.
   2. Proclamations can be issued by a governor or a mayor. In many areas, a mayor or governor can issue a proclamation without action from the city council or state legislature.
   3. A letter requesting a proclamation should follow the same format used to write a federal official (see VI. Communicating with elected officials). Within the text of the letter, include:
      a. The reason for the proclamation (e.g., Kidney Disease Awareness and Education Week, Nephrology Nurses Week).
      b. How the issue affects local citizens.
      c. A fact sheet with statistics and trends for your state or city that relate to the issue (these statistics can provide the text of the proclamation). For example: The number of patients with ESRD in the state, the number of new cases each year, the number of nurses caring for these patients. Individual state fact sheets are available on the ANNA website at http://www.annanurse.org/advocacy/state-health-policy/state-fact-sheets
      d. Dates of the proclamation.
   4. Always follow up with a written thank-you note.
   5. Inform the ANNA National Office of the proclamation.

VI. Communicating with elected officials.

A. Can it make a difference?
   1. The offices of elected officials count all calls, emails, faxes, and mail received.
   2. The staffers log each opinion that is expressed.
   3. The information is then reported to the member of Congress.

B. Effective communication with legislators is the backbone of every successful legislative initiative.

C. All representative offices handle communication differently; consider contacting your members' offices to inquire about their preferred method of communication (ANNA, 2013a).

D. Legislators rely on informed citizens to help them identify key issues and positions on those issues. Nephrology nurses are the experts who have personally seen the devastating effects of kidney disease on patients and their families.

E. Phone calls.
   1. Plan what you want to say before you call.
   2. Always be polite.
   3. Ask to speak to the staff member who handles the issue you wish to discuss.
   4. Begin by identifying yourself by name and as a registered nurse.
   5. Find out the member's position on an issue. It can be a waste of time for the member if they already support your position.
   6. Keep the call brief; make a few brief points.
      a. State your position.
      b. Be clear and specific as to what you are asking your representative to do (e.g., support or cosponsor the legislation).
   7. Be prepared to answer questions and leave a telephone number where you can be contacted to provide additional information.
   8. Offer assistance to the member or staff.
   9. Express appreciation.
   10. Always send a follow-up letter.

F. Sending a letter or email.
   1. Guidelines are the same for state and federal officials.
   2. Do your homework; have a clear and concise message. Identify exactly what you want, when

you want it, and who you want it from (Mason et al., 2007).

3. Standard mail takes quite a while longer. Since the anthrax attacks in 2001, the U.S. Postal Service mail has been handled differently by Congress. If your message is time sensitive, consider email, fax, or phone communication.
4. Addressing the letter or email (Smith, 2006).
   a. Senator.
      (1) The Honorable (full name)
      United States Senate
      Washington, DC 20510
      (2) Dear Senator:
   b. House of Representatives.
      (1) The Honorable (full name)
      United States House of Representatives
      Washington, DC 20515
      (2) Dear Congressman/Congresswoman: *or* Dear Representative:
   c. Committee chair.
      (1) Use examples above for address.
      (2) Dear Mr. Chairman/Dear Madam Chairwoman:
5. Text of the letter.
   a. Concisely state purpose of letter in first paragraph.
   b. State your name and identify yourself as a registered nurse.
   c. Include your area of work and define the patients you care for.
   d. Give your full home mailing address so the office can verify you are a constituent and send you a response. If you are not a constituent, identify any connection with the recipient's district (e.g., working in the district).
   e. Identify legislation by HR____ or S____.
   f. Be very specific as to what you would like your representative to do.
   g. Include vital pieces of information such as how this issue affects the member's constituents. If applicable, make it personal. Relay personal testimony or experiences.
   h. Offer assistance to serve as a resource to the member or the staff.
   i. Express appreciation for the time and effort the member has spent or will spend on the issue or bill.
   j. Request a response from the member.
   k. Overall tips (ANNA, 2013a).
      (1) Keep text to one page.
      (2) Address only one issue per letter.
      (3) Be honest and accurate.
      (4) Be brief and to the point.
6. Be sure to follow up.
   a. By phone or with another letter.
   b. If you receive an unsatisfactory response, write or call again.
      (1) Express appreciation for the time and effort.
      (2) Be firm and polite in communicating your position.
      (3) Review the vital pieces of information.
7. Keep in regular contact.

G. Scheduling a visit with a representative.
   1. Guidelines are the same for Washington, DC, or your local district.
      a. Remember you do not need to go to Washington, DC, to see your representatives.
      b. Visit the district office; it is probably very near your home.
      c. Plan your visit carefully.
   2. Contact the representative's scheduler or secretary by phone or email.
      a. Washington, DC, switchboard.
         (1) House: (202) 225-3121
         (2) Senate: (202) 224-3121
      b. The district office will be listed in the blue pages of your local telephone book.
      c. State your name and where you live.
      d. State that you are a registered nurse.
      e. Relay the reason for requesting a visit to speak with the member.
      f. The scheduler may ask for a faxed request. In that case, create a concise letter with all the necessary information (refer to previous information on composing the letter).
      g. Include a list of those who would like to attend the meeting.
      h. You will be notified by phone or email of the appointment time.
      i. Be polite and persistent.
      j. Call or re-fax a request if there is no response from the scheduler within a week of your initial contact.

H. Meeting your elected official.
   1. The visit may be with the member or his/her staff.
   2. Role playing is a good method to prepare for the visit.
   3. Be on time, preferably early, for your appointment.
   4. Be prepared to wait for the member or staff.
      a. It is not uncommon for a member to be late.
      b. If you are interrupted, take the opportunity to continue your meeting with the staff.
   5. Introduce yourself with confidence.
      a. For example: "Hello, I'm Jane Doe, and I'm a registered nurse in your district."
      b. Hand the member your business card and deliver a firm handshake.
   6. Be flexible; the meeting may have to take place in a hallway or common area.

7. Organize objectives for the visit (Smith, 2006).
   a. Be clear in what you want to achieve.
   b. Clarify your key points.
   c. Bring any materials that support your position.
      (1) Members are required to take positions on many issues.
      (2) Members may lack the information about the pros and cons of an issue.
      (3) Concise handouts also provide useful information for review after you leave.
8. Assign a spokesperson if multiple people are attending.
9. Explain how the issue impacts the member's constituency. Provide a personal story or example.
10. Provide concise information on a one-page document or have a packet of information to leave with the member.
11. Always be polite and listen carefully.
12. Be prepared to answer questions. If you do not know the answer to a question, be honest and say so. Offer to supply the information.
13. Offer to assist the member regarding your issue.
    a. Become a resource on kidney disease for your elected official. A well informed nephrology nurse can be a valued resource to an elected official and their staff (ANNA, 2013a).
    b. If requested, be prepared to supply additional information.
14. Express appreciation.
15. Enjoy the visit!
    a. Do not be nervous. You are the expert in the care of patients with kidney disease.
    b. You are building a long-term relationship with your elected official.
16. After the visit.
    a. Keep notes as a reference for the next time you visit your member.
    b. Send a thank-you note either written or faxed.
       (1) Be sure to briefly review the key points of your issue.
       (2) Send any additional information that was requested.
    c. Share the result of the meeting with the local ANNA chapter.
17. Maintain communication with the member both in Washington and the home district.

I. Locating your members of Congress.
   1. http://www.annanurse.org, Click on Advocacy and then Take Action (CapWiz)
   2. http://www.senate.gov
   3. http://www.house.gov
   4. http://www.firstgov.org
   5. http://www.congress.org
   6. http://thomas.loc.gov

VII. Impacting factors in healthcare policy.

A. General.
   1. Economic environment: Rising healthcare costs and diminishing resources plays an increasing role in the ability of nurses to provide care to patients.
   2. Variable quality/health disparities.
   3. Nursing shortage: In addition to the pressures of the shortage, nurses are impacted by downsizing, long work hours, work place injuries and burdensome documentation processes taking the nurse away from the bedside (Mason et al., 2007). Nursing shortages have been linked to increased mortality, staff violence, injuries, cross infection, and adverse post-op events (Collins-McNeil et al., 2012).
   4. Safe work practices.
      a. Safe patient handling and mobility.
      b. Needle safety.
      c. Environmental health.
      d. Disaster preparedness and response.
      e. Healthy work environments.
   5. Patient safety: impacted by the economic environment, healthcare environment, proliferation of new technology and the need for the acceptance of healthcare providers' recognition that they do make mistakes (Mason et al., 2007).
   6. Aging nursing workforce (Collins-McNeil et al., 2012).
      a. The average age of the nurse in 2010 was over 45.
      b. Nursing requires extreme physical demands and aging nurses are reported to have higher workload demands than in other professions.
      c. Increased workloads, challenging work environments, and new technologies also increase the risk of stress, injury, and decreased health.
      d. As the aging nursing workforce retires, there is a concern about a lack of qualified nurses and the impact on patient outcomes.
      e. Nursing challenges:
         (1) Retain knowledgeable, skilled nurses.
         (2) Aggressively recruit younger nurses.
         (3) Develop initiatives to retain nurses.
         (4) Minimize physical demands.
            (a) Reduce ergonomic risk factors: work station redesign to avoid bending and twisting.
            (b) Restructure job duties and tasks to match the skill set of each worker.
            (c) Provide flexible hours, ensuring regular breaks.
            (d) Perform job safety analyses.
   7. Evidence-based practice: process by which scientific evidence is used to improve health care and specific patient outcomes to determine the

appropriate deployment of resources (Mason et al., 2007).

B. Patient Protection and Affordable Care Act (ACA): Signed into law in 2012, the provision designed to expand access to insurance, increase consumer protections, emphasize prevention and wellness, improve quality and system performance, expand the health workforce, and curb rising healthcare costs (National Conference of State Legislatures, 2011).
  1. Effective January 1, 2014.
  2. Key provisions (National Conference of State Legislatures, 2011).
     a. Requires employers to cover workers or pay penalty, expectations for small employers. Penalties will be assessed in 2015.
     b. Provides tax credits to certain small business to cover identify costs for health insurance, beginning tax year 2010.
     c. Provides individuals to have insurance with some exceptions. Penalties will be assessed in 2015.
     d. Provides creation of state based (or multistate) insurance exchanges to help individuals and small businesses purchase insurance.
        (1) Varies between states.
        (2) Covers 10 essential health benefits categories.
     e. Federal subsidies limit premium costs to 2% of income for those at 133% of federal poverty guidelines, increasing to 9.5% of income for those who earn between 300% and 400% of poverty guidelines.
     f. Expanded Medicaid coverage to those with incomes below 133% of federal poverty guidelines.
     g. Created temporary high-risk pools for those who cannot purchase insurance on the private market due to pre-existing conditions, beginning July 1, 2010.
     h. Provided insurance plans to cover young adults on parents' policies, beginning September 23, 2012.
     i. Established a national, voluntary long-term care insurance program for "community living assistance services and supports" (CLASS), regulations were issued October 1, 2012.
     j. Enacted consumer protections to enable people to retain their insurance coverage, beginning 2010:
        (1) Prohibits lifetime monetary caps on insurance coverage and limits use of annual caps.
        (2) Prohibits insurance plans from excluding coverage for children with pre-existing conditions.
        (3) Prohibits insurance plans from canceling coverage, except in cases of fraud.
        (4) Establishes state based rate review for "unreasonable" insurance premium increases.
        (5) Establishes an office of health insurance consumer assistance or an ombudsman program.
        (6) Establishes the share of premiums dedicated to medical services.
  3. Additional Insurance Reforms, effective January 1, 2014.
     a. Prohibit most insurance plans from excluding people with pre-existing conditions and discriminating based on health status.
     b. Impose annual monetary caps on coverage.
     c. Reforms that require guaranteed issues and renewal of policies, premium rating rules, nondiscrimination in benefits and mental health and substance abuse parity.
  4. Created the Center for Medicare and Medicaid Innovation (CMMI).
     a. CMMI was established by section 1115A of the Social Security Act, as added by section 3021 of the Affordable Care Act.
     b. With CMS, CMMI supports the testing of innovative healthcare payment and service delivery models to reduce program expenditures while preserving or enhancing the quality of care. Additional information can be found on their website at http://innovation.cms.gov
  5. Nursing's role. Opportunities for advanced practice registered nurses (APRNs) (ANA, 2012): only about half of all private insurers currently credential and directly reimburse APRNs, creating a barrier in the existing insurance marketplace. There is an opportunity to educate policymakers about the importance of using APRNs to ensure consumers access to high quality, cost-effective care.

C. Accountable Care Organizations (ACOs).
  1. ACOs: established by the ACA, final rules were released on November 2, 2011 (CMS, 2013a).
     a. What are they?
        (1) ACOs are groups of physicians, hospitals, and other healthcare providers who voluntarily provide coordinated high quality care to the Medicare patients they serve.
        (2) The goal is to provide high quality care while spending healthcare dollars wisely and share in the savings it achieves for the Medicare program.
        (3) Through coordinated care, patients, including the chronically ill, will get the right care at the right time, avoiding

unnecessary duplication of services and the prevention of medical errors.

b. There are several ACO programs including:
   (1) The Medicare Shared Savings Program: for fee-for-service beneficiaries; provides incentives for ACOs that meet standards for quality performance and reduce costs while putting patients first.
   (2) Advance Payment ACO Model: Designed for physician-based and rural providers. Through this model, selected participants will receive upfront and monthly payments, which they can use to make investments in their care coordination infrastructure.
   (3) Pioneer ACO (CMS, 2012).
      (a) A Center for Medicare & Medicaid Services (CMS) Innovation Center initiative designed to support organizations with experience operating as an ACO.
      (b) The Pioneer ACO Model was to test the impact of different payment arrangements in helping the organizations achieve the goals of providing better care to patients while reducing Medicare costs.
      (c) Designed for organizations with experience offering coordinated, patient-centered care and operating in ACO-like arrangements. Through an open competitive process, 32 organizations were selected.
      (d) This 3-year model, began January 1, 2012, is different from the Shared Savings Program, based on the payment model.

2. Comprehensive ESRD Care Model or ESRD Seamless Care Organizations (ESCOs) (CMS, 2013b).
   a. Designed to test and evaluate a new model of payment and care delivery specific to Medicare beneficiaries with ESRD.
   b. Participating organizations will consist of groups of healthcare providers, led by healthcare providers experienced in the care of ESRD beneficiaries. Organizations must include representation from dialysis facilities, nephrologists and other Medicare providers and suppliers (e.g. durable medical equipment suppliers, ambulance providers, drug or device manufacturers). Each ESCO must have at least:
      (1) One dialysis facility and one independent nephrologist or nephrology group practice as a participation owner in the ESCO.
      (2) The governing body of the ESCO must include at least one patient representative or independent consumer advocate.
   c. To be eligible, ESCOs must have a minimum of 350 beneficiaries "matched" to their organization.
   d. Participating organizations will be clinically and financially responsible for all care offered to a group of matched beneficiaries, not limited to dialysis care. Services could include primary/preventive care, vascular access, specialty care, etc.
   e. Set quality measures will be used to assess both health and experience for beneficiaries.
   f. CMS will assess performance in improving outcomes; ESCOs that succeed in offering high quality care that lowers the total cost will have the opportunity to share in the Medicare savings with CMS.

Part 4. Learning Opportunities for Nurses in Health Policy

I. General (Mason et al., 2007).

A. Programs and courses in schools of nursing.

B. Degree programs in public health, public administration, and public policy.

C. Continuing education programs: nursing organizations, state nursing organizations, American Association of Retired Persons, Women's League of Voters.

D. Volunteer service: work on a political campaign.

II. Organizational and national programs for nurses.

A. ANNA's Health Policy Workshop.
   1. Sponsored by ANNA and held every other year in Washington, DC.
   2. All interested ANNA members are invited to attend. Also in attendance are the members of the Health Policy Committee and the Board of Directors.

B. Nurse in Washington Internship (NIWI).
   1. Sponsored by Nursing Organizations Alliance, held annually in Washington, DC.
   2. ANNA has supported, provided representation, and provided faculty since the first program in 1985.

C. Robert Wood Johnson Health Policy Fellowship Program.
   1. Sponsored by the Institute of Medicine of the National Academies.
   2. These hands-on internships offer experience in policy making in Washington, DC, with a member of Congress.
   3. More information can be found at http://www.healthpolicyfellows.org/fellowship_howtoapply.php

D. White House Fellowship Program.
   1. Hands-on experience for young professionals to experience policy making in the highest levels of the federal government.
   2. More information can be found at http://www.whitehouse.gov/about/fellows/

References

Abood, S. (2007). Influencing health care legislative arena. *The Online Journal of Issues in Nursing, 12*(1), Manuscript 2. Retrieved from http://www.nursingworld.org/MainMenuCategories/ANAMarketplace/ANAPeriodicals/OJIN/TableofContents/Volume122007/No1Jan07/tpc32_216091.aspx

American Nephrology Nurses' Association (ANNA). (2012). *ANNA legislative handbook. Pitman, NJ*: Author. Retrieved from http://www.annanurse.org/sites/default/files/download/reference/health/handbook.pdf

American Nephrology Nurses' Association (ANNA). (2013a). *ANNA health policy toolkit*. Retrieved from http://www.annanurse.org/download/reference/health/hpToolkit.pdf

American Nephrology Nurses' Association (ANNA). (2013b). *ESRD education week: Planning and orientation guide*. Retrieved from http://www.annanurse.org/events/kidney-disease-awareness-and-education-week/planning-and-orientation

American Nephrology Nurses' Association (ANNA). (2013c). *Overview: Brief history of Medicare end stage renal disease (ESRD) reimbursement*. Retrieved from http://www.annanurse.org/download/reference/health/esrdReimbursementFactSheet.pdf

American Nurses Association (ANA). (2001). *Code of ethics for nurses*. Retrieved from http://nursingworld.org/MainMenuCategories/EthicsStandards/CodeofEthicsforNurses/Code-of-Ethics.pdf

American Nurses Association (ANA). (2012). *State health insurance exchanges: The critical role of nurses & nursing*. Retrieved from http://nursingworld.org/MainMenuCategories/Policy-Advocacy/Positions-and-Resolutions/Issue-Briefs/State-Health-Insurance-Exchanges.pdf

Centers for Medicare & Medicaid Services (CMS). (2012). *Pioneer accountable care organization model: General fact sheet*. Retrieved from http://innovation.cms.gov/Files/fact-sheet/Pioneer-ACO-General-Fact-Sheet.pdf

Centers for Medicare & Medicaid Services (CMS). (2013a). *Accountable care organizations (ACOs): General information*. Retrieved from http://innovation.cms.gov/initiatives/ACO/.

Centers for Medicare & Medicaid Services (CMS). (2013b). *Comprehensive ESRD care model fact sheet*. Retrieved from http://www.cms.gov/Newsroom/MediaReleaseDatabase/Fact-sheets/2014-Fact-sheets-items/2014-04-15.html

Collins-McNeil, J., Sharpe, D., & Benbow, D. (2012). Aging workforce: Retaining valuable nurses. *Nursing Management, 43*(3), 50-54.

Gallup. (2012). *Honesty/ethics in professions*. Retrieved from http://www.gallup.com/poll/1654/Honesty-Ethics-Professions.aspx

Kuchta, K., Gilbreth, A., Gilman. C., & Wieler, A. (2006). The legislative process and the kidney care quality and improvement act of 2005. *Nephrology Nursing Journal, 2*(33), 229-232.

Mason, D., Leavitt, J.K., & Chaffee, M.W. (2002). *Policy and politics in nursing and health care* (4th ed.). St. Louis: Mosby.

National Council of State Boards of Nursing. (2013). *Nursing licensure compact*. Retrieved from https://www.ncsbn.org/nlc.htm

National Conference of State Legislatures. (2011). *The affordable care act: A brief summary*. Retrieved from http://www.ncsl.org/portals/1/documents/health/hraca.pdf

Smith, K. (2006). Public policy issues and legislative process. In A. Molzahn & E. Butera (Eds.), *Contemporary nephrology nursing: Principles and practice* (2nd ed., pp. 833-850). Pitman, NJ: American Nephrology Nurses' Association.

Swaminathan, S., More, V., Mehrotra, R., & Trivedi, A. (2012). Medicare's strategy for end stage renal disease now embraces bundled payment and pay-for-performance to cut costs. *Health Affairs, 31*(9), 2051-2058.

Ulrich, B. (2011). Patient advocacy is job one. *Nephrology Nursing Journal, 5*(38), 391.

United States House of Representatives. (n.d.). *Main page*. Retrieved from http://www.house.gov

United States Senate. (n.d.). *Main page*. Retrieved from http://www.senate.gov

CHAPTER 4

Essentials of Disaster and Emergency Preparedness in Nephrology Nursing

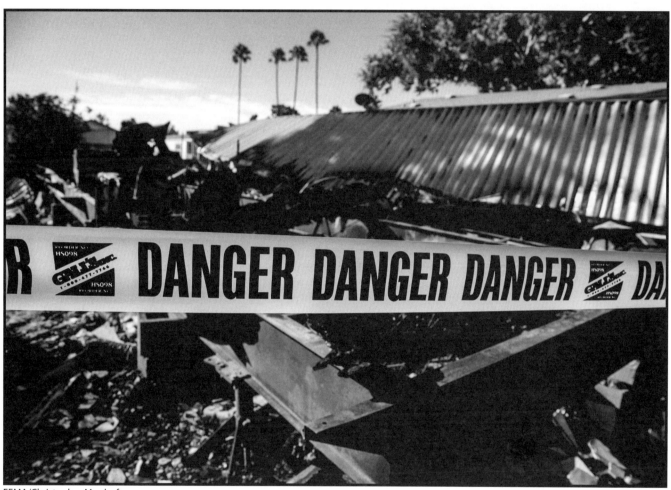

FEMA/Christopher Mardorf

Chapter Editor and Author
Norma Gomez, MSN, MBA, RN, CNN

CHAPTER **4**

Essentials of Disaster and Emergency Preparedness in Nephrology Nursing

This offering for **1.9 contact hours** is provided by the American Nephrology Nurses' Association (ANNA).

American Nephrology Nurses' Association is accredited as a provider of continuing nursing education by the American Nurses Credentialing Center Commission on Accreditation.

ANNA is a provider approved by the California Board of Registered Nursing, provider number CEP 00910.

This CNE offering meets the continuing nursing education requirements for certification and recertification by the Nephrology Nursing Certification Commission (NNCC).

To be awarded contact hours for this activity, read this chapter in its entirety. Then complete the CNE evaluation found at **www.annanurse.org/corecne** and submit it; or print it, complete it, and mail it in. Contact hours are not awarded until the evaluation for the activity is complete.

Example of reference for Chapter 4 in APA format. One author for entire chapter.

Gomez, N. (2015). Essentials of disaster and emergency preparedness in nephrology nursing. In C.S. Counts (Ed.), *Core curriculum for nephrology nursing: Module 1. Foundations for practice in nephrology nursing* (6th ed., pp. 109-137). Pitman, NJ: American Nephrology Nurses' Association.

Interpreted: Chapter author. (Date). Title of chapter. In …

Cover photo by Christopher Mardorf /FEMA. Napa, CA, August 30, 2014 – Fire damage from broken gas lines at the Napa Valley Mobile Home Park in the City of Napa, California, which was struck by a 6.0 earthquake at 3:20 a.m. on August 24. 2014. At least 103 structures (44 homes, 59 businesses) were tagged "RED" by inspectors as unsafe to enter in the City of Napa after the earthquake. FEMA supports state, local, and tribal governments in their efforts to recover from the effects of natural disasters.

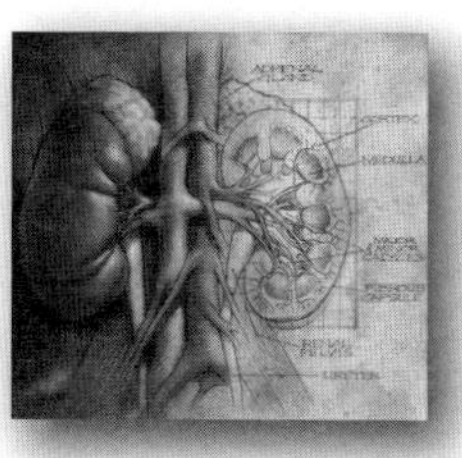

CHAPTER 4

Essentials of Disaster and Emergency Preparedness in Nephrology Nursing

Purpose

The purpose of this section is to review the different types of natural and man-made disasters, provide strategies for formulating a plan for individual facilities, provide a general outline for developing a facility Disaster Preparedness Plan, and provide guidance in coordinating drills. Any disaster preparedness plan requires the collaboration of administration, clinical and technical staff, patients, families, state, federal, and community resources.

Objectives

Upon completion of this chapter, the learner will be able to:

1. Define the role of the nephrology nurse in disaster and emergency preparedness and response.
2. Provide strategies for training of employees, patients, and communities in disaster emergency preparedness.
3. Identify best practices and strategies for dealing with disaster situations.

SECTION A
General Disaster Plan

I. Introduction.

A. A disaster can be defined as a significant disruption to the health and safety of a community caused by natural forces, physical failures of machinery or infrastructures, or the conduct of an individual(s) that results in a significant disruption of health and safety of the community or the nation (ANA, 2002). Disasters, natural and otherwise, are unpredictable and occur with regularity. CMS (2008) defines an emergency as "a situation requiring help or relief, usually created by an unexpected event" (p. 2).

B. In the past 40 years, more than 6,000 documented natural disasters have affected more than 5 billion people. These, along with man-made disasters, take a toll on thousands of lives, with a cost of billions of dollars.
   1. Natural disaster examples.
      a. Hurricane Sandy (2012).
      b. Haiti earthquake (2010).
      c. Hurricane Katrina (2005).
      d. Asian Tsunami (2004).
      e. Hurricane Andrew (1992).
      f. Oakland Wildfires (1991).
      g. Hurricane Hugo (1989).
      h. Loma Prieta earthquake (1989).
      i. Hurricane Camille (1969).
   2. Man-made examples.
      a. Workplace violence.
      b. School violence.
      c. Chemical explosions.
      d. Terrorist attacks (e.g., 9/11 in 2001).

C. Disasters do not need to be a large-scale global event.
   1. The majority will occur on a local level affecting a defined community.
   2. Specific emergency preparedness procedures should be developed for different kinds of emergencies. Each facility should assess their local area and region for potential risks of particular emergencies (e.g., coastal areas for hurricanes and flooding).
   3. Man-made disasters such as power outages, fuel or water supply failures, chemical spills, arson, and other disasters should also be considered. Once the risks are identified, a comprehensive, systemic emergency preparedness program should be developed which outlines concrete goals, identifiable resources, education, and communication of the plans.

4. Facilities not directly affected by the disaster may become "surge" facilities. The patients will be directed to the unaffected facility for treatment. The surge of patients may surpass the existing resources. Facilities should have policies and procedures for receiving an overflow of patients that may or may not have their dialysis or insurance information. The Kidney Community Emergency Response Coalition (KCER), the Networks, and larger providers may be able to assist with deploying additional staff to the "surge" facilities.

D. Know and meet requirements federal, state, and local requirements.
  1. Conditions for Coverage (CfC)§ 494.60. The conditions for coverage outline specific requirements for disaster planning for dialysis facilities.
    a. The dialysis facility must develop and implement emergency preparedness policies and procedures, risk assessment, and the communication plan based on the emergency plan set forth in the CfC.
    b. The policies and procedures must be reviewed and updated at least annually.
    c. Education and training of staff and patients, including drills.
    d. Staff training must be provided and evaluated at least annually and be such as to ensure that staff can demonstrate knowledge of emergency procedures, including informing patient of:
      (1) What to do.
      (2) Where to go, including instructions for occasions if evacuated.
      (3) Whom to contact if an emergency occurs while the patient is not in the dialysis facility.
      (4) Provide alternate emergency phone number for the facility.
      (5) Emergency disconnect procedures. Don't forget your home patients when you do your drills.
      (6) Ensure that, at a minimum, patient care staff maintain current CPR certification.
      (7) Ensure that nursing staff are properly trained in the use of emergency equipment and emergency drugs.
    e. Medical records need to include evidence of education in emergency evacuation and emergency preparedness, including some measure of patient understanding, such as return teaching or demonstration.
    f. Both patients and staff need to be encouraged to develop personal emergency plans.
      (1) It is important to review these plans at a staff meeting so everyone is aware of each other's needs.
      (2) Encourage patients, including patients dialyzing at home and transplant recipients, to develop a personal plan.
    g. When preparing for a hurricane, the facility may bring in all the patients for treatment, but remember the staff also needs to prepare their home and family. The staff schedule should have some overlap so staff can leave and prepare their homes.
    h. Evaluate the effectiveness of emergency and disaster plans at least annually and update them as necessary.
  2. The Joint Commission.
    a. Mandates all healthcare facilities create a plan for emergency preparedness.
    b. Practice the plan twice a year.

E. It is important to have a written disaster plan outlining the steps to be taken.
  1. Make the plan easy to understand and accessible to all personnel and patients.
  2. Evaluate and update the plan at least annually.
  3. Facilities should coordinate the plan with community resources: sister units, local hospitals, and local emergency management offices.
    a. Sister units should be at least 50 miles from your facility. (Sister units are facilities where there is an agreement to dialyze the affected patients when the facility is no longer operational.)
    b. Local hospitals, in some communities, are identified as command centers to facilitate communication with staff and patients.
    c. Local emergency management offices and local disaster management agencies must be contacted at least annually to ensure that such agency is aware of dialysis facility needs in the event of an emergency.
      (1) There must be documented evidence of this contact.
      (2) Educate local emergency management on the presence of the dialysis facility and patients in their area.

F. The emergency management model created by the Federal Emergency Management Agency (FEMA) can be used as a basis for any disaster preparedness program (http://ww.fema.gov). The model is a continuous process with four activity phases. This model emphasizes evaluation and applying lessons learned to future events.
  1. *Preparedness phase* involves developing a plan to educate the workforce and other stakeholders.
  2. *Response phase* occurs when the plan is implemented. The important components of this phase are patient management and communication.

3. *Recovery phase* encompasses intervention to get the community back to the pre-disaster baseline.
4. *Mitigation stage* involves activities undertaken to minimize the negative impact of the event.

II. General disaster plans.

A. Included in this section is a general disaster plan that can be used for all types of disasters. It uses a basic three-phase process: pre-event planning, response to the event, and post-event restoration (Lettieri, 2006). Specific actions for each type of natural and man-made disaster are outlined in the various sections below. No matter what the disaster may be and what type of plan is developed, you must always address communication, water, power, supplies, transportation, and safety issues.

B. Fortunately, many disasters can be predicted days ahead of time: hurricanes and, to some extent, wildfires, blizzards, ice storms, and floods. Advance warning and early evacuation will likely improve the safety of patients on dialysis during disasters.

Orderly pre-disaster evacuation of patients on dialysis contributes greatly to ensuring continuity of medical care. Evacuees may travel on their own to stay with friends or in hotels, or they may travel by private car, public transportation, redeployed school buses, and other means to predesignated shelter sites.

Healthcare providers should help patients develop individualized evacuation plans that address particular issues, including lack of transportation, limited financial/social support, and physical and psychological factors (Kopp et al., 2007).

1. Community evacuation centers are categorized into two types: general population shelters and special-needs shelters.
   a. Special needs shelters are designed to accommodate evacuees (and their family members) who require assistance with activities of daily living (e.g., patients with dementia and mobility limitations), specific medical needs that require intervention by health professionals (e.g., oxygen, glucose monitoring, dressing changes, medication administration), and infectious diseases that require protective equipment or isolation.
   b. The specific criteria for admitting patients to special-needs shelters are set by each state. States differ as to whether patients on dialysis are sent to general population shelters or special-needs shelters.
   c. Community evacuation shelters may be staffed by local, state, and federal emergency response personnel, as well as by volunteers.
2. The Conditions for Coverage requires centers to implement processes and procedures to manage medical and nonmedical emergencies likely to threaten the health or safety of patients, staff, or the public, including fire, equipment or power failures, care-related emergencies, water supply interruption, and natural disasters likely to occur in the facility's geographic area. Centers should also prepare for other types of emergencies that are identified after the performance of a facility risk assessment.
3. Establish emergency admission and treatment procedures that include:
   a. Contact information.
   b. Insurance information.
   c. Physician orders.
   d. Treatment history.
   e. Lab results.

III. Pre-event.

The pre-event phase is defined by anticipation, planning, and training. The focus on this phase is to decrease risks associated with events.

A. Review possible threats to the facility. The disaster plan must address all potential threats including but not limited to:
1. Susceptibility to hurricanes, floods, tornadoes, earthquakes, wild fires, and volcanic eruptions.
2. Man-made disasters such as power outages, water main breaks, fuel and water supply, chemical spills, arson, bomb threat.
3. Chemical plant or nuclear power plant accidents.

B. Communication is a critical component (see Table 4.1).
1. Existing communication systems should be assessed: cell phones, ham radios, satellite phones, toll-free numbers, TV and radio public service announcements, local newspapers, and websites.
2. An analog phone must be available (newer phones require electricity to work).
3. Identify communication needs.
   a. Purchase or rent satellite phones.
   b. Train staff on use of each device.
4. Depending on the type of event, identify "who" will have the responsibility of communicating damage of the facility before, after, and during the event.
5. As part of the disaster plan, distribute multiple keys and alarm codes to the building.
6. Communicate status of the facility. Possible methods include:
   a. Sign on front door of clinic to inform patients and staff where to report.
   b. Staff member staying at facility to communicate the plan (dependent on type of disaster).
   c. Prearranged destination if facility not operational.
   d. Media announcements.

Table 4.1

Disaster Communications Template

Normal Status	Level I	Level II	Level III	Level IV
Normal Operations – Preparations	**Potential Threat Identified – Monitoring Phase**	**Disaster Event Identified as Threat**	**Imminent Threat**	**Post-event/Recovery**
Education	**Monitor situation**	**Activate emergency team**	**Activate at facility level**	**Coordinate and respond**
This includes patients, employees, and physicians. Includes diaster plans, personal preparedness, emergency diet, local hazards, etc.	Monitor local news/weather, EOCs, network, etc., concerning expected conditions.	Team responsible for emergency coordination and preparation.	Team responsible for emergency coordination and preparation. Review plan and post-event procedures.	Team responsible for emergency coordination and recovery.
Update contact information	**Education**	**Conference calls**	**Conference calls**	**Conference calls**
Patients, employees, and physicians. Local and out-of-town.	This includes patients, employees, and physicians. Includes disaster plans, personal preparedness, emergency diet, local hazards, etc.	Calls with primary team concerning threatened event preparation; include physicians in planning.	Calls with primary team concerning threatened event preparation, include physicians in planning.	Calls with primary team concerning event recovery, facility status, assistance needed, etc., and include physicians.
Supplies	**Update contact information**	**Post-closure signage**	**Update closure signage**	**Update closure signage**
Order and maintain 2 weeks of treatment supplies. During extreme weather "seasons," additional supplies should be on hand as physical plant allows.	Patients, employees, and physicians. Local and out-of-town.	Ensure signs with facility emergency contact and alternate treatment information are posted on front door.	Ensure signs with facility emergency contact and alternate treatment information are posted on front door.	Ensure signs with facility emergency contact and alternate treatment information are posted on front door.
Facility policy and procedures	**Facility policy and procedures**	**Communicate status to network/EOC**	**Communicate status to network/EOC**	**Communicate status to network/EOC**
Review policy and procedures. Ensure all employees are familiar.	Review and discuss policy and procedures. Ensure all employees are familiar.	Advise facility status/operational plan to network, transportation providers, and local Emergency Operations Center (EOC).	Update facility status/operational plan to network, transportation providers, and local Emergency Operations Central (EOC).	Advise facility status (damage, operations, special needs, etc.) to network, transportation providers, and local EOC.
Meetings	**Inventory**	**Inventory**	**Inventory**	**Inventory**
Schedule meetings with physicians, local EOCs, hospitals, LDOs, etc., to discuss disaster preparedness and planning.	Review inventory to ensure 2 weeks of treatment supplies on hand. Update if necessary. Communicate with contracted supply vendors regarding contingency deliveries.	Verify inventory includes 2 weeks of additional supplies on hand at facility. Update if necessary.	Verify inventory includes 2 weeks of additional treatment supplies on hand. Make adjustments where necessary.	Assess inventory of treatment supplies on hand and update if necessary. Activate appropriate contingency plans with contracted vendors for deliveries.
Local hazards	**Local hazards**	**Local hazards**	**Local hazards**	**Local hazards**
Be familiar with flood zones and evacuation areas.	Be familiar with flood zones and evacuation areas.	Be familiar with flood zones and evacuation areas.	Evaluate evacuation areas and prepare to activate plan.	Be familiar with flood zones and evacuation areas, damage areas and curfews in effect.

Normal Status	Level I	Level II	Level III	Level IV
Normal Operations – Preparations	**Potential Threat Identified – Monitoring Phase**	**Disaster Event Identified as Threat**	**Imminent Threat**	**Post-event/Recovery**
Home/Family preparedness	**Home/Family preparedness**	**Home/Family preparedness**	**Home/Family preparedness**	**Home/Family preparedness**
Encourage patients and employees to prepare their home and family for potential event.	Encourage patients and allow employees time to prepare their home and family (gas, extra money, generators, etc.).	Encourage patients and verify that employees have prepared their home and families (gas, extra money, generators, etc.). Allow additional time necessary to complete preparations.	Encourage patients and verify that employees have prepared their home and families (gas, extra money, generators, etc.). Allow additional time necessary to complete preparations.	Assess damage/status of employees, physicians, and patients, and coordinate and assist where identified.
Special needs	**Special needs**	**Special needs**	**Special needs**	**Special needs**
Identify the special needs of patients, employees, and physicians.	Identify the special needs of patients, employees, and physicians.	Identify the special needs of patients, employees, and physicians.	Reassess the special needs of patients, employees, and physicians.	Identify the special needs of patients, employees, and physicians.
Communication plan	**Communication plan**	**Staffing needs**	**Staffing needs**	**Staffing needs**
Establish a call-tree, call-down, voicemail, or call system for key facility people. Identify how facility status and plans are communicated to staff and patients.	Review call-tree, call-down, voicemail, or call system for key facility people. Identify how facility status and plans are communicated to staff and patients.	Evaluate staffing needs and adjust schedules relative to threatened event.	Evaluate staffing needs and adjust schedules relative to threatened event.	Evaluate staffing needs and adjust schedules for post-event.
Physical plant	**Physical plant**	**Physical plant**	**Physical plant**	**Physical plant**
Evaluate needs to protect property and continuous operations. Agreements with local contractors, electricians, fuel, etc.	Evaluate needs to protect property and continuous operations. Agreements with local contractors, electricians, fuel, etc.	Evaluate needs to protect property and continuous operations. Agreements with local contractors, electricians, fuel, etc.	Prepare facility for event; may include boarding/shuttering, securing medical records in waterproof containers, covering machines/equipment/computers, backup data, generator, securing biohazardous waste, extra keys to key people, etc.	Evaluate facility status before allowing personnel into facility. Determine needs for reestablishing operations. Ensure water and equipment safety. Outside hazards (trees, down power lines, building damage).
Update contact information	**Update contact information**	**Update contact information**	**Update contact information**	**Update contact information**
Maintain updated contact information on patients, employees, and physicians – local and out-of-town.	Verify contact information on patients, employees, and physicians – local and out-of-town. Ask about evacuation plans.	Verify contact information on patients, employees, and physicians – local and out-of-town. Ask about evacuation plans.	Reverify contact information on patients, employees, and physicians – local and out-of-town. Ask for final evacuation plans.	Verify contact information on patients, employees, and physicians – local and out-of-town, current location (shelter, home, family, etc.).
Medical and employment records	**Medical and employment records**	**Medical and employment records**	**Medical and employment records**	**Locate**
Upon admission/employment, and in coordination with facility policies thereafter, issue patient/staff ID badges, facility emergency contact info, curfew letters, and emergency contact cards.	Confirm that employees and patients can locate ID badges, facility emergency contact info, curfew letters, and emergency contact cards.	Confirm that employees and patients have located ID badges, facility emergency contact info, curfew letters, and emergency contact cards. Reissue if necessary.	Instruct employees and patients to maintain ID badges, facility emergency contact info, curfew letters, and emergency contact cards on their person at all times.	Locate and account for all of your patients, employees, and physicians — local and out-of-town (shelter, home, family, etc.). Notify network of any missing patients from your facility and/or evacuees treated at your facility.

e. Use of toll-free numbers.
f. Network office.
7. Always have a battery-operated backup radio available.
8. Routinely update contact numbers for staff, patients, community resources, and vendors.
a. If possible, before the event, determine where patients and staff will be during or after the storm: at their own home, with a relative in town, with relative out of town, shelters, etc.
b. Inform shelters of the special dietary and fluid needs of the dialysis patient as well as their priority status for transportation to a dialysis facility when conditions are clear to travel.

C. Water, power, and supplies are essential considerations.
1. Identify emergency shut-off valves (electrical, gas, water, fire alarm, security, etc.).
2. There may be a "boil water advisory" issued by the community.
a. Review water treatment components and assess ability to perform dialysis treatments.
b. Increase testing procedures for microbial assessment.
3. Municipal water suppliers may "shock" (hyperchlorinate) their systems to regain acceptable bacterial levels for drinking water. Review and update testing procedures for potential chlorine/chloramine breakthrough.
4. Locate emergency lighting in the patient care area, water treatment area, and along the path of egress.
5. Assess the potential need for generator.
a. Determine the size of the generator needed to run essential equipment.
b. Determine what equipment will be running with the generator.
c. Identify sources for purchasing or renting a generator if needed post-disaster.
d. If using a generator:
(1) Develop maintenance schedules and perform maintenance according to manufacturer's operating manual.
(2) Assess fuel needs. Assume at least 2 to 3 days of fuel.
(3) Determine where the fuel is to be stored.
(4) Make arrangements for a contract for fuel before the event takes place.
(5) Develop a plan to protect the generator before, during, and after the disaster.
(6) Install an electrical transfer switch or automatic bus transfer (ABT).
(7) Make arrangement for security to protect the generator(s) and fuel from theft during and after the event.
6. Keep at least a 2-week additional inventory during times an event may occur (e.g., for hurricane season it would be in summer; for winter storms it would be in winter). Remember that the reprocessing of dialyzers will probably not be performed during a disaster. Provide enough dry packs to perform treatments.
7. Put in place an agreement with a water vendor for delivery of water needs. Some facilities have agreements with local fire departments to supply water after an event.
8. Disposal of "spent dialysate" may be an issue, especially with flooding (Counts, 2001).

D. Transportation for patients and staff.
1. If the facility has elevators, make an alternate plan for transporting the patients to the treatment area.
2. As part of the facility plan, include contracts with local transportation companies for patient transportation before and after the event.
3. Depending on the nature of the event (e.g., flooding, mudslides, icy roads), consider alternate methods for staff transportation.
4. If the disaster results in major damage/destruction to a community, pay attention to law enforcement requirements to enter the affected area. Curfews may be instituted affecting patients, staff, and physicians.

E. Hazardous waste disposal: develop a plan for alternate disposal of hazardous waste.

F. Electronic medical records.
1. Back up records prior to the threat.
2. If server is off-site, ensure remote access to records.

G. Include emergency standing orders in each patient's medical record regarding changes in their prescription during a disaster.

IV. Response to the threat – execution of the plan.

A. Communication is critical in this phase. Plans must include coordination of:
1. Setting up a command center.
2. Placing a poster in the facility door stating where patients and staff are to report.
3. Informing patients and staff of the TV/radio stations that will announce facility closures.
4. Advertising toll-free numbers to be used at specific times post-event.
5. Contacting state board of nursing.
a. To assess what tasks can be performed by an out-of-state RN or LPN in the case of a federally declared emergency.
b. If not part of the Nurse Licensure Compact (NLC), develop a process to obtain temporary licensure for nonstate nurse volunteers.

B. Implementation of the 3-Day Emergency Diet Plan.
  1. Ensure copies of the 3-Day Emergency Diet Plan are available for distribution.
  2. If the facility does not have an emergency diet plan, refer to the National Kidney Foundation website (http://www.kidney.org). Patients should receive education on the emergency diet plan prior to implementation.

C. Triage.
  1. Before and after an event, patients may need additional treatments.
  2. If the facility was damaged, sister facilities may be dialyzing these patients. This influx of additional patients could require a change in the patient's schedule and prescribed therapy, such as decreased hours in treatment or increase in the length of time between treatments.
  3. The medical director or attending physician must give orders for any changes to a patient's dialysis prescription.

V. Post-event phase restoration.

A. Assess the facility structure before bringing patients back to the facility for treatment.

B. Implement a process for locating patients and staff. Contact the local ESRD Networks and CMS for assistance.

VI. Lessons learned.

A. Report to work during a disaster.
  1. All nurses must be prepared to report to work during a disaster. Studies have shown that the most common barriers to a healthcare worker's ability to report to work during an emergency are transportation and child, elder, and pet care obligations, while the most frequently cited barriers to willingness are fear and concern for one's self and their family (Qureshi et al., 2005).
  2. Each nurse should have a family emergency plan that is reviewed with all family members and a personal emergency plan that delineates the steps to be taken to assure that family obligations are provided for in the event he or she is called upon for emergency work.
  3. The most inclusive information for family emergency planning has been developed by the Department of Homeland Security (DHS).
     a. Found under the "Ready America" tab at http://www.ready.gov
     b. On the site, find a checklist for emergency supply kits, suggestions for developing and recording a family plan, and tips to become informed about one's own community disaster plans and warning systems.

B. Posttraumatic stress.
  1. Defined as emotional reactions. May include feelings of shock, fear, grief, resentment, guilt, shame, helplessness, hopelessness, confusion, memory loss, and interpersonal relationship issues (NCTSN & PTSD, 2007). It can take 2 to 4 weeks for symptoms to develop.
  2. Early intervention includes psychological first aid, psychological debriefing, and crisis counseling by a mental health professional.
  3. Basic objectives.
     a. Enhance immediate and ongoing safety, and provide physical and emotional comfort.
     b. Help survivors articulate immediate needs and concerns, as well as gather additional information as appropriate.
     c. Connect survivors as soon as possible to social support systems, including family members, friends, neighbors, and community resources.

C. Administrative processes may be interrupted: billing and payroll.
  1. Develop an alternative plan to deliver payroll if normal process is disrupted.
  2. Identify an alternative billing process if normal process is disrupted.
  3. Know your lease: Who is responsible for repairing the facility damage?
  4. List of administrative resources (e.g., attorney, risk manager).

D. Provide patients with a waterproof container that contains last treatment sheet, dialysis prescription, and facility contact information. Also include current hepatitis B vaccination status and documentation of TB testing.

E. Institute a form of patient identification such as an armband, name badge, etc.

SECTION B
Natural Disasters

I. Hurricanes.

A. A hurricane is an intense tropical weather system with a well-defined circulation and maximum sustained winds of 74 mph (64 knots) or higher.
  1. A tropical depression is a weather system with rotating winds of 38 mph (33 knots) or less.
  2. Tropical storms have sustained winds of 39 to 74 mph (34 to 63 knots) and these systems are "named" according to a list developed by the

National Hurricane Center. In the Western Pacific, hurricanes are called typhoons. Similar storms in the Indian Ocean are called cyclones.
3. Hurricanes are identified by categories and range from I to V.
   a. A category I storm has winds from 74 to 95 mph with storm surges from 4 to 5 feet.
   b. A category V has winds over 155 mph and storm surges higher than 18 feet.
4. The Saffir-Simpson Hurricane scale describes a hurricane's intensity (see Table 4.2).
   a. Additional information can be found on the National Oceanic and Atmospheric Administration (NOAA) website, http://www.nhc.noaa.gov
   b. Government and businesses use this information to estimate potential flooding and potential property damage when the hurricane makes landfall.

B. Hurricane facts.
1. The United States shoreline attracts large numbers of people from Maine to Texas with an estimated 45 million people living along the hurricane-prone shoreline.
2. Hurricane season extends from the first of June to the end of November with peak months being August and September.

C. Hurricane warning system.
1. Effective in providing timely warnings for people to properly prepare or move inland when a hurricane is threatening the area.
2. It is becoming more difficult to evacuate the coastal areas due to the increased population and the summer tourist seasons.
3. People are still complacent and delay taking action, causing increased property damage and loss of life.

D. Hurricane watch.
1. During this advisory, closely monitor the NOAA weather station.
2. As appropriate, the staff should be allowed to leave in shifts to fuel cars and prepare homes and secure cash, home supplies, and medications.
3. Initiate facility disaster plan. Advise patients to begin personal preparations.

E. Hurricane warning.
1. During this advisory, monitor NOAA weather station for updates.
2. Continue following established disaster plan.
   a. Bring all outside items inside or tie down securely.
   b. Confirm that the facility has a battery-operated phone to continue phone service.
   c. Ensure facility has storm shutters or other approved window protection.
   d. If facility has a generator, ensure enough fuel is safely stored and is available to run the generator.

F. After the storm.
1. Everyone who must drive should do so carefully, avoiding dangling wires and flooded areas.
2. Report damaged water, sewer, and electric lines to the authorities.
3. Assess the possible presence of gas leaks.

G. Facility action plan.
1. During a hurricane, homes, businesses, public buildings, roads, and power lines may be damaged by high winds and flooding. Debris can break windows and doors. Roads and bridges can be washed away by flash flooding or blocked by debris. The force of the wind alone can topple trees, remove roofs, and undermine weakened buildings. In addition, hurricanes can spawn tornadoes, which add to the destruction.
2. Risk assessment should include the following:
   a. Facility.
      (1) Assess for potential loss of power, water, phone.
      (2) Assess potential flooding.
      (3) Check roof for potential leaks or damage.
      (4) Check windows for potential leaking.
   b. Supplies and equipment.
      (1) Increase supply inventory during hurricane season.
      (2) Ensure equipment (including backups) are in operating order and will be secure during the storm.
   c. Medical records.
      (1) Store all medical records in protective coverings.
      (2) Place them at least 24 inches off the floor.
      (3) Ensure electronic medical records have off-site access.
   d. Community.
      (1) Assess emergency response, special shelters, and transportation for patients and staff.
      (2) Make sure facility has a battery-operated backup radio.
   e. Roles of staff members.
      (1) Review chain of command procedures.
      (2) Ensure staff has time to secure their own home by thorough scheduling.
   f. Patient education and preparation.
      (1) Educate patients on in-center, peritoneal dialysis and patients at home regarding disaster plan.

Table 4.2

Hurricane Categories

Category	Winds	Storm Surge	Damage
I	74–95 mph	4–5 ft	No real damage to buildings. Damage primarily to unanchored mobile homes, shrubbery, and trees. Minor coastal flooding and pier damage.
II	96–110 mph	6–8 ft	Considerable damage to shrubbery, trees, signs, roofing, doors, and windows. Considerable mobile home damage and unprotected small crafts.
III	111–130mph	9–12 ft	Structural damage to small residences, large trees blown down, mobile homes destroyed.
IV	131–155 mph	13–18 ft	Complete roof failures, shrubs, trees, sign damage, complete destruction of mobile homes. Extensive damage to windows and doors.
V	> 155 mph	> 18 ft	Complete roof failure on residences and industrial buildings. Small utility buildings blown over or blown away. Severe extensive damage to windows and doors.

Based on information from National Hurricane Center, http://nhc.noaa.gov

   (2) Transplant recipients should be part of the transplant program's plan.
3. Communication.
   a. Review and evaluate contact information to ensure it is still accurate for staff, patients, emergency contacts, and community resources.
   b. Perform drills to give staff hands-on preparation of what to do, to familiarize them with their role, and to identify potential problems with the plan.
   c. Keep all members of the team informed of the progress of any tropical storm or hurricane. Administrative personnel should meet when a storm is expected and make a final assessment of the plan and initiate a specific plan of action.
   d. Ensure all patients are dialyzed prior to the storm with an understanding they may need to go 3 days without dialysis. Notify transportation companies of the schedule change.
   e. Develop a communication plan in the event phones are not functioning.
      (1) Include the use of cell phones, satellite phones, ham-operated radios.
      (2) Coordinate with sister facilities, local hospitals, and local, state, and federal agencies.
      (3) Contact the local Emergency Operations Center (EOC) to inform them of your facility's status.
      (4) Contact American Red Cross regarding potential need for shelters.
      (5) Coordinate facility information and patient tracking with the ESRD Network.
      (6) Use identified local radio and TV stations to get information out to the patients regarding opened and closed facilities.
4. Patients on in-center hemodialysis.
   a. Establish strategies to ensure transportation agencies can facilitate transportation post-event.
   b. Must be able to perform emergency disconnect procedures in case power outage occurs during treatment.
5. Patients on home hemodialysis.
   a. Should have a 2-week supply of dialysis supplies in case shipments are delayed.
   b. Must be able to perform emergency disconnect procedures in case power outage occurs during treatment.
   c. Patients should register with local water and power company for priority reinstatement of services.
   d. If electrical power or water service is interrupted, patients must know how to contact the dialysis staff so that alternate dialysis arrangements can be made.
6. Patients on peritoneal dialysis.
   a. An electrical outage will affect continuous cycling peritoneal dialysis (CCPD) patients.

These patients should possess the ability to perform manual exchanges during these times.
   b. If patients are unable to perform as many exchanges as ordered, they should have instructions to implement the emergency diet and fluid restrictions plan.
   c. Patients on peritoneal dialysis should have an emergency 5-day supply of antibiotics for potential peritonitis.
   d. Should report their status post-event to the facility.

7. Transplant recipients.
   a. Patients should keep and carry with them a current list of their medications and have a 2-week supply on-hand.
   b. Should report their status post-event to the transplant center.
8. Patients with diabetes.
   a. Should keep extra insulin and syringes.
   b. Should keep extra batteries for glucometer.
9. Acute programs. Usually one of the staff members stays at the hospital during the storm and is then relieved after the storm.
10. All patients should:
   a. Keep and carry a current list of medications.
   b. Keep a 2-week supply of their medications.
   c. Wear a medical information emblem.
   d. Have a battery-powered AM/FM radio and flashlight with extra batteries.
   e. Have a list of emergency phone numbers.
   f. Prepare themselves and their household in the same ways as the general public.

H. Post-event.
   1. Assess damage and determine when treatments can resume.
   2. Become aware of any imposed curfews.
   3. Locate and contact patients and staff as soon as possible post-event.
   4. Staff and patients should have proper identification to be allowed into disaster area.

II. Tornadoes.

A. Tornadoes are violent storms that develop from powerful thunderstorms, or they can accompany tropical storms and hurricanes as the systems move onto land.
   1. Appear as rotating, funnel-shaped clouds that extend from a thunderstorm to the ground with whirling winds that can reach 300 miles per hour.
   2. Can last up to 1 hour, but most last less than 10 minutes. Occasionally, tornadoes develop so rapidly that little, if any, advance warning is possible. Before a tornado hits, the wind may die down and the air may become very still. A cloud of debris can mark the location of a tornado even if a funnel is not visible.
   3. Generally occur near the trailing edge of a thunderstorm. It is not uncommon to see clear, sunlit skies behind a tornado.

B. Tornado facts.
   1. In the United States, the National Weather Service issues tornado forecasts nationwide.
   2. Annually 1,000 tornadoes are reported across the United States, resulting in approximately 70 deaths each year. Most deaths are the result of flying or falling debris.
   3. Every state is at risk for tornadoes.
   4. Peak tornado seasons.
      a. Southern Plain – May to early June.
      b. Gulf Coast – early spring.
      c. Northern Plains and upper Midwest – June and July.
      d. East of the Rocky Mountains – spring and summer months.
      e. Southern States – March through May.
      f. Northern States – late spring through early summer.
   5. Though tornadoes may move in any direction, the average tornado moves southwest to northeast.
   6. Tornadoes can occur at any time but most frequently occur between 3 and 9 p.m.

C. Tornado watch.
   1. Conditions are right for a tornado to form in the next several hours.
   2. During a tornado watch, staff and patients should stay tuned to radio or television weather reports. They need to be aware of changing weather conditions.

D. Tornado warning.
   1. Indicates that a tornado has been spotted or indicated by weather radar.
   2. Indicates imminent danger to life and property to those in the path of the storm.
   3. Take immediate safety precautions.
      a. Quickly get to a designated tornado safe area.
      b. Safe areas are away from windows and glass.
      c. Take cover within 1 minute of a tornado warning. Sixty-two percent of those killed by tornadoes die in the first 5 minutes after a warning is issued.
      d. Do not open windows.
      e. Do not use elevators.

E. Facility Action Plan.
   1. Devise a mechanism to receive and monitor weather reports.
   2. Know emergency alerts signals (sirens, etc.).

3. After the tornado.
   a. Locate and contact patients and staff as soon as possible post-event.
   b. Check for injured or trapped persons.
   c. Provide first aid when appropriate.
   d. Contact authorities.
   e. Take caution for potential fires and hazards like broken electrical wires, water leaks, and gas or oil leaks. Have proper tools available to turn off these valves if necessary to do so.
4. Evacuate patients if necessary.
5. Patient education and preparation.
   a. Inform patients of the designated tornado safe place.
   b. Review procedures and perform drills for emergency discontinuation of the dialysis treatment.
   c. Instruct patients to lie face down and protect their head and dialysis access (as possible).
   d. If patients miss a dialysis treatment, they should start the emergency diet plan.
   e. Patients need to inform shelter personnel about special needs such as diet and transportation issues.
6. Patients on in-center hemodialysis.
   a. If patients are dialyzing in the facility, remove them from treatment using emergency disconnect protocols. Move or assist patients into the designated safe area.
   b. If moving cannot be accomplished, move them away from windows. Place them under sturdy furniture and cover with blanket, coats, pillows, etc.
   c. Instruct patients to protect their head and dialysis access extremity.
7. Patients on home hemodialysis.
   a. Must be able to perform emergency disconnect procedures.
   b. The patient and partner should go to safe area in lowest area of the house.
   c. The dialysis access and the person's head should be protected.
   d. The patient needs to get under a strong bench or heavy furniture if possible.
   e. Patients residing in a mobile home must be able to get out of the mobile home quickly and take shelter in a building with a strong foundation.
   f. If shelter is not available, instruct the patient to lie in a ditch or low-lying area between the tornado and mobile home.
   g. Instruct patients to register with local water and power company for priority reinstatement of services.
   h. Patients must know how to contact the dialysis staff so that alternate dialysis arrangements can be made if there is a loss of power and/or water.
8. Patients on peritoneal dialysis.
   a. An electrical outage will affect patients on continuous cycling peritoneal dialysis. These patients should possess the ability to perform manual exchanges during these times.
   b. If patients are unable to perform as many exchanges as ordered, instruct them to implement the emergency diet and fluid restrictions plan.
   c. Patients on peritoneal dialysis should have an emergency 5-day supply of antibiotics for potential peritonitis.
   d. Patient should be aware of emergency procedures to follow for tornadoes (see E.7. Patients on home hemodialysis).
   e. When possible, they need to contact the facility to report their status.
   f. Instruct patients to register with local water and power company for priority reinstatement of services.
   g. Patients must know how to contact the dialysis staff so that alternate dialysis arrangements can be made if there is a loss of power and/or water.
9. Transplant recipients.
   a. Patients should keep and carry a current list of their medications and have a 2-week supply on hand.
   b. When possible they need to contact the transplant center to report their status.
   c. Patient should be aware of emergency procedures to follow for tornadoes (see E.7. Patients on home hemodialysis).
10. Patients with diabetes.
    a. Keep extra insulin and syringes.
    b. Keep extra batteries for glucometer.
    c. Patient should be aware of emergency procedures to follow for tornadoes (see E.7. Patients on home hemodialysis).
11. All patients should:
    a. Keep and carry a current list of medications.
    b. Keep a 2-week supply of their medication.
    c. Wear a medical information emblem.
    d. Have a battery-powered AM/FM radio and extra batteries and a flashlight with batteries.
    e. Have a list of emergency phone numbers.
    f. Prepare themselves and their household the same ways as the general public.

III. Floods.

A. All floods are not alike. Some floods develop slowly, occasionally over a period of days.
   1. Flash floods are usually caused by slow-moving thunderstorms or thunderstorms that move over the same area one after the other.
   2. Overland flooding occurs outside a defined river or stream, such as when a levee is breached, but can still be destructive.

3. Everyone needs to be aware of flood hazards no matter where they live, but particularly those who live in low-lying areas, near water or downstream from a dam.
4. Even very small streams, gullies, creeks, culverts, dry streambeds, or low-lying ground that appears harmless in dry weather can flood.
5. Every state is at risk for this hazard.

B. Flood facts.
   1. Every year, devastating floods occur throughout the United States.
      a. 90% of all presidentially declared natural disasters involve flooding.
      b. In the United States, an average of 200 people lose their lives annually, and flood damage averages more than $6 billion (USGS, 2006).
      c. The majority of deaths from flooding occur when people become trapped in automobiles that stall while driving through flooded areas. Nearly half of all flood fatalities are vehicle-related.
   2. Floodwater often contains infectious organisms, including intestinal bacteria such as *E. coli*, salmonella, shigella, hepatitis A virus, and agents of typhoid, paratyphoid, and tetanus.
      a. Signs and symptoms experienced by the victims of waterborne microorganisms are similar, even though they are caused by different pathogens.
      b. Symptoms include nausea, vomiting, diarrhea, abdominal cramps, muscle aches, and fever.
      c. Most cases of sickness associated with flood conditions are brought about by ingesting contaminated food or water.
      d. Tetanus, however, can be acquired from contaminated soil or water entering broken areas of the skin, such as cuts, abrasions, or puncture wounds. Tetanus is an infectious disease that affects the nervous system and causes severe muscle spasms. The symptoms may appear weeks after exposure and may begin as a headache, but later develop into difficulty swallowing or opening the jaw.
   3. Floodwaters also may be contaminated by agricultural or industrial chemicals or by hazardous agents present at flooded hazardous waste sites.
      a. Flood cleanup crew members who must work near flooded industrial sites may be exposed to chemically contaminated floodwater.
      b. Different chemicals cause different health effects, but the signs and symptoms most frequently associated with chemical poisoning are headaches, skin rashes, dizziness, nausea, excitability, weakness, and fatigue.
   4. Pools of standing or stagnant water become breeding grounds for mosquitoes, increasing the risk of encephalitis, West Nile Virus, or other mosquito-borne diseases.
   5. The principal causes of flooding in the Eastern United States and the Gulf Coast are hurricanes and storms.
   6. The principal causes of floods in the Western United States are snowmelts and rainstorms.
   7. Flooding is the only natural disaster for which the Federal government provides insurance: FEMA's National Flood Insurance Program.

C. Flood watch.
   1. A flood is possible in the area.
   2. Stay alert to signs of flash flooding and be ready to evacuate on a moment's notice.
   3. Flash flood watch indicates that flash flooding is a possibility in or close to the watch area.
      a. Those in the affected area are urged to be ready to take action if a flash flood warning is issued or flooding is observed.
      b. These watches are issued for flooding that is expected to occur within 6 hours after heavy rains have ended.

D. Flood warning.
   1. Flooding is already occurring or will occur soon in the area.
   2. Listen to local radio and TV stations for information and advice.
   3. If told to evacuate, do so as soon as possible.
      a. Do not drive around barricades — they are there for everyone's safety.
      b. If a car stalls in rapidly rising waters, it should be abandoned immediately and the person(s) should climb to higher ground.

E. Facility Action Plan.
   1. Develop a mechanism to receive and monitor weather reports.
   2. Know local emergency alert signals.
   3. Install sump pumps with backup power.
   4. A licensed electrician should raise electric components (switches, sockets, circuit breakers and wiring) at least 12 inches above the facility's projected flood elevation.
   5. Install backflow valves or plugs for drains, toilets, and other sewer connections to prevent floodwaters from entering.
   6. Turn off all main utilities at the main power switch, and close the main gas valve if evacuation appears necessary.
   7. After the flooding.
      a. All patients and staff should be accounted for.
      b. Evacuate patients from the area if necessary.
      c. Patients and staff should have immunization

records available or be aware of last tetanus shot, in case of contamination during or after the flood.

8. Patient education and preparation.
   a. Inform patients where to go if forced to evacuate.
   b. Periodically review procedures and drills for the emergency termination.
   c. If patients will have to miss a dialysis treatment, implement the emergency diet and fluid restriction plan.
   d. Patients need to tell shelter personnel about their special needs, such as diet and transportation to and from dialysis treatments.
9. Patients on in-center hemodialysis.
   a. If patients are dialyzing in the facility, stop the treatment using emergency protocols.
   b. Move patients into the designated safe area. Provide physical assistance as needed.
10. Patients on home hemodialysis.
    a. Must be able to perform emergency disconnect procedures.
    b. The patient and partner should go to a safe area in highest part of the house.
    c. Should register with local water and power company for priority reinstatement of services.
    d. If electrical power or water service is interrupted, they must know how to contact the dialysis staff to make alternate dialysis arrangements.
11. Patients on peritoneal dialysis.
    a. An electrical outage will affect patients on continuous cycling peritoneal dialysis. These patients should possess the ability to perform manual exchanges during these times.
    b. If patients are unable to perform as many exchanges as ordered, instruct them to implement the emergency diet and fluid restrictions plan.
    c. Patients on peritoneal dialysis should have an emergency 5-day supply of antibiotics for potential peritonitis.
    d. Patient should be aware of emergency procedures to follow for floods (see E.10. Patients on home hemodialysis).
    e. Contact the facility to report their status.
    f. Patients should be instructed to register with local water and power company for priority reinstatement of services.
    g. Patients must know how to contact the dialysis staff to make alternate dialysis arrangements if there is a loss of power and/or water.
12. Transplant recipients.
    a. Keep and carry a current list of medications and have a 2-week supply on hand.
    b. Contact the transplant center to report their status, when possible.
    c. Should be aware of emergency procedures to follow for floods (see E.10. Patients on home hemodialysis).
13. Patients with diabetes.
    a. Should keep extra insulin and syringes.
    b. Should keep extra batteries for glucometer.
    c. Should be aware of emergency procedures to follow for floods (see E.10. Patients on home hemodialysis).
14. All patients.
    a. Keep and carry a current list of medications.
    b. Keep a 2-week supply of medication.
    c. Wear a medical information emblem.
    d. Have a battery-powered AM/FM radio and flashlight with extra batteries.
    e. Have a list of emergency phone numbers.
    f. Prepare themselves and their household the same ways as the general public.

IV. Winter storms and blizzards.

A. A winter storm is defined as a storm with heavy snow and/or ice, sustained winds or wind gusts up to 35 miles per hour or greater, and considerable falling or blowing snow.

B. Winter storm facts.
   1. The National Weather Service refers to winter storms as the "deceptive killers" because most deaths are indirectly related to the storm.
      a. People die in traffic accidents on icy roads.
      b. Hypothermia occurs from prolonged exposure to cold, especially in the very young and elderly.
         (1) Watch for signs of hypothermia: uncontrollable shivering, memory loss, disorientation, incoherence, slurred speech, drowsiness, and apparent exhaustion.
         (2) If you detect symptoms of hypothermia, get the patient to a warm location, remove wet clothing, warm the center of the body first and give warm, nonalcoholic beverages if the patient is conscious.
         (3) Get medical help as soon as possible.
      c. Watch for signs of frostbite.
         (1) Signs include loss of feeling and white or pale appearance in extremities such as fingers, toes, ear lobes, and the tip of the nose.
         (2) If symptoms are detected, get medical help immediately.
         (3) Asphyxiation occurs related to improper use of fuels with power outages.
   2. Power outages are typically caused by ice forming on power lines and pulling the lines down and or breaking the poles.

a. Outages can last 1 to 10 days (usually 3 days).
b. Most local government agencies do not supply generators to homes or businesses.

C. Winter storm watch.
1. A winter storm with heavy snow and/or ice is possible in your area.
2. Warnings are usually issued 24 to 48 hours in advance of the storm.
3. Listen to NOAA Weather Radio or local stations for updated information.
4. Prepare for a potential storm.
   a. Review the disaster plan.
   b. Educate patients and staff of the actions to be taken in the event of a winter storm or blizzard.
   c. Make sure patients are aware of emergency diet plans if dialysis is not possible as scheduled.
5. Changes in temperature, snowfall, and wind can occur quickly.
6. Avoid unnecessary travel.

D. Winter storm warning.
1. A winter storm is occurring or will soon occur.
2. Initiate disaster plan.

E. Blizzard warning.
1. Sustained winds or wind gusts up to 35 miles per hour or greater and considerable falling or blowing snow.
2. Visibility is reduced to less than ¼ mile.
3. Expected to prevail for a period of 3 hours or longer.

F. Ice storm.
1. Freezing rain or drizzle creating danger to trees and power lines and on roads.
2. Stay indoors and dress warmly.
3. Listen to radio or television (have battery-operated radios available).

G. Facility Action Plan.
1. Policies and procedures to guide emergency response.
   a. Make sure there is a mechanism to receive and monitor weather reports.
   b. Because traffic accidents are the leading cause of death during winter storms, advise patients not to attempt to go out or drive until the storm is over and the roads are clear.
   c. If patients are dialyzing when a blizzard hits, have a plan for them to stay until the storm is over and the roads are clear.
   d. If patients have to miss a dialysis treatment, instruct them to begin their emergency meal plan.
   e. If patients have to go to a shelter, they should notify someone from the facility.
2. Patient education and preparation.
   a. Consider conducting educational days in the autumn related to winter storm preparedness. Include diet planning, shopping lists, shelter information, safety tips, etc.
   b. Winter storms may cause clinic closures or inability for patients to arrive for dialysis treatments.
3. Patients on in-center dialysis. Review procedures patients need to follow if their regularly scheduled dialysis treatments are interrupted.
4. Patients on home hemodialysis.
   a. Keep a 2-week supply of dialysis supplies in case deliveries are delayed.
   b. Register with local water and power company for priority reinstatement of services.
   c. Know emergency discontinuation of procedures in case power outage occurs during their treatment.
   d. If electrical power or water service is interrupted, they must know how to contact the dialysis staff to make alternate dialysis arrangements.
5. Patients on peritoneal dialysis.
   a. An electrical outage will affect patients on continuous cycling peritoneal dialysis. These patients should possess the ability to perform manual exchanges.
   b. If patients are unable to perform as many exchanges as ordered, instruct them to implement emergency diet and fluid restriction plan.
   c. They should keep a 2-week supply of peritoneal dialysis supplies in case delivery of supplies is delayed.
   d. Patients on peritoneal dialysis should have an emergency 5-day supply of antibiotics for potential peritonitis.
6. Transplant recipients.
   a. Keep at least a 2-week supply of immunosuppressive medication on hand in case they are unable to get to the pharmacy.
   b. When possible, they need to contact the transplant center to report their status.
7. Patients with diabetes.
   a. Keep extra insulin and syringes.
   b. Keep extra batteries for glucometer.
8. All patients.
   a. Keep and carry a current list of medications.
   b. Keep a 2-week supply of medication.
   c. Wear a medical information emblem.
   d. Have a battery-powered AM/FM radio and flashlight with extra batteries.
   e. Have a list of emergency phone numbers.
   f. Prepare themselves and their household the same ways as the general public.

V. Earthquakes.

A. An earthquake is the sudden, rapid shaking of the earth, caused by the breaking and shifting of subterranean rock as it releases strain that has accumulated over a long time.

B. Earthquake facts.
  1. All 50 states and five U.S. territories are at some risk for earthquakes.
  2. Earthquakes can happen at any time of the year.
  3. Earthquakes occur suddenly and without warning.
    a. Can seriously damage buildings.
    b. Disrupt gas lines, electric, and telephone service.
    c. Trigger landslides, floods, and tsunamis.
    d. Aftershocks may occur for weeks after the initial earthquake.

C. Facility Action Plan.
  1. Facility inspection by a structural engineer.
    a. Have a contract with an engineering firm to assess safety of building after earthquake.
    b. All storage selves should be braced and have "lips."
    c. Place large or heavy objects on lower shelves.
    d. Store breakable items such as bottled foods and glass in low, closed cabinets with latches.
    e. Use safety glass.
    f. Secure heavy equipment to the floor.
    g. Ensure dialysis machine wheels are always in the locked position except when moving.
  2. Develop an evacuation plan.
    a. Designate "gathering" area after the quake away from buildings.
    b. If patients are dialyzing when an earthquake occurs, instruct them to remain calm and seated until instructed otherwise by staff. Face them away from any windows.
    c. Stay inside until the shaking stops and it is safe to go outside. Do not exit a building during the shaking. Research has shown that most injuries occur when people inside buildings attempt to move to a different location inside the building or try to leave.
    d. Locate and contact patients and staff as soon as possible post-event.
  3. If patients have to miss a dialysis treatment, instruct them to begin their emergency diet and fluid restriction plan.
  4. If patients have to go to a shelter, they should notify the facility.
  5. Patients on in-center dialysis.
    a. Prepare for aftershocks.
    b. Check for injuries; give first aid if needed.
    c. Remove patients from the machine if deemed appropriate.
    d. Determine if any structural damage.
    e. Evacuate if deemed appropriate.
    f. Review procedures patients need to follow if their regularly scheduled dialysis treatments are interrupted.
  6. Patients on home hemodialysis.
    a. Must keep hemodialysis machine wheels locked at all times.
    b. Keep a 2-week supply of dialysis supplies in case deliveries are delayed.
    c. Should register with local water and power company for priority reinstatement of services.
    d. Must know emergency disconnect procedures in case power outage occurs during treatment.
    e. If electrical power or water service is interrupted, they must know how to contact the dialysis staff to make alternate dialysis arrangements.
  7. Patients on peritoneal dialysis.
    a. Ensure patients keep CCPD equipment wheels locked at all times.
    b. An electrical outage will affect patients on continuous cycling peritoneal dialysis. These patients should possess the ability to perform manual exchanges.
    c. If patients are unable to perform as many exchanges as ordered, instruct them how to implement emergency diet and fluid restriction plan.
    d. Keep a 2-week supply of peritoneal dialysis supplies in case delivery of supplies is delayed.
    e. Patients on peritoneal dialysis should have an emergency 5-day supply of antibiotics for potential peritonitis.
  8. Transplant recipients.
    a. Keep at least 2-weeks supply of immunosuppressive medication on hand in case they are unable to get to the pharmacy.
    b. When possible, recipents need to contact the transplant center to report their status.
  9. Patients with diabetes.
    a. Keep extra insulin and syringes.
    b. Keep extra batteries for glucometer.
  10. Acute dialysis patients. There may be increased hospital admissions and need for acute treatments due to crush injuries.
  11. All patients.
    a. Keep and carry a current list of medications.
    b. Keep a 2-week supply of medication.
    c. Wear a medical information emblem.
    d. Should have a battery-powered AM/FM radio and flashlight with extra batteries.
    e. Should have a list of emergency phone numbers.

f. Prepare themselves and their household the same ways as the general public.

12. After the earthquake, inspect utilities.
    a. Check for gas leaks. If you smell gas or hear blowing or hissing noise, open a window and quickly leave the building.
        (1) Turn off the gas at the outside main valve if you can and call the gas company.
        (2) If you turn off the gas for any reason, it must be turned back on by a professional.
    b. Look for electrical system damage.
        (1) If you see sparks or broken or frayed wires, or if you smell hot insulation, turn off the electricity at the main fuse box or circuit breaker.
        (2) If you have to step in water to get to the fuse box or circuit breaker, call an electrician first for advice.
    c. Check for sewage and water lines damage.
        (1) If you suspect sewage lines are damaged, avoid using the toilets and call a plumber.
        (2) If water pipes are damaged, contact the water company and avoid using water from the tap.
        (3) Ensure water meets AAMI requirements prior to resuming treatments in the facility.

VI. Fires and wildfires.

A. Smoke from wildfires is a mixture of gases and fine particles from burning trees and other plant materials.

B. Fire facts.
1. Each year more than 2,500 people die and 12,600 are injured in home fires in the United States.
2. In just 2 minutes, a fire can become life-threatening. In 5 minutes, a residence can be engulfed in flames (FEMA, 2013).
3. Smoke can cause coughing, scratchy throat, irritated sinuses, shortness of breath, chest pain, headaches, stinging eyes, and runny nose. In people who have heart or lung disease, smoke triggers or worsen symptoms.
4. Smoke may worsen symptoms for people who have pre-existing respiratory conditions, such as respiratory allergies, asthma, and chronic obstructive pulmonary disease (COPD). Symptoms may include inability to breathe normally, cough with or without mucus, chest discomfort, wheezing, and shortness of breath.
5. Pay attention to local air quality reports.
    a. Listen and watch for news or health warnings about smoke.
    b. Find out if the community provides reports about the Environmental Protection Agency's Air Quality Index (AQI).
    c. Pay attention to public health messages about taking additional safety measures.
    d. Refer to visibility guides if available. Not every community has a monitor to measure the number of particles that are in the air. In the western part of the United States, some communities have guidelines to help people estimate AQI based on how far they can see.
6. If persons are advised to stay indoors, indoor air should be kept as clean as possible.
    a. Keep windows and doors closed unless it is extremely hot outside.
    b. Run an air conditioner if available, but keep the fresh-air intake closed and the filter clean to prevent outdoor smoke from getting inside.
    c. If an air conditioner is not available and it is too warm to stay inside with the windows closed, seek shelter elsewhere.
7. Dust masks are not enough.
    a. Paper "comfort" or "dust" masks, commonly found at hardware stores, are designed to trap large particles such as sawdust. These masks will not protect your lungs from smoke.
    b. For more information about effective masks, see the Respirator Fact Sheet on the Center for Disease Control (CDC) National Institute for Occupational Safety and Health website, http://www.cdc.gov

C. Facility Action Plan.
1. Perform routine life, fire, and safety inspections. Identify two ways to get out of each room. The dialysis facility must comply with applicable provisions of the 2000 edition of the Life Safety Code of the National Fire Protection Association.
2. Maintain appropriate placement, quantity, and type of fire extinguishers.
3. Train staff in the use of fire extinguishers.
4. Develop and use policies and procedures for handling and storing flammables.
5. Develop, communicate, and enforce smoking policies for patients, staff, and visitors.
6. Devise procedures for informing the fire department of the facility's location and determination of approximate response time.
7. Institute procedures for activating the fire alert system.
8. Involve staff and patients in performing emergency dialysis discontinuation drills.
    a. Drills should include evacuation procedure, use of fire extinguishers, and shut-off valves for electricity, water, and gas.
    b. Drills should be evaluated and reported to supervisory personnel.
9. Learn about the history of wildfires in your area.
    a. Be aware of weather; long periods without rain increase the risk of wildfires.

b. If considering evacuation, check the condition of the roads.
c. Eliminate brush, trees, and other vegetation to create a safety zone. This area should be approximately 30 feet from the building.
d. Encourage patients and staff to create safety zones around their houses.

10. Locate and contact patients and staff as soon as possible post-event.

VII. Mudslides.

A. Landslides occur when masses of rock, earth, or debris move down a slope. Debris flows, also known as mudslides, are a common type of fast-moving landslide that tends to flow in channels.

B. Mudslide facts.
1. Landslide causes.
   a. Disturbances in the natural stability of a slope.
   b. Accompany heavy rains or follow droughts, earthquakes, or volcanic eruptions.
   c. Develop when water rapidly accumulates in the ground and results in a surge of water-saturated rock, earth, and debris.
   d. Usually start on steep slopes and can be activated by natural disasters.
   e. Areas where wildfires or human modification of the land have destroyed vegetation on slopes are particularly vulnerable to landslides during and after heavy rains.
2. In the United States, landslides and debris flows result in 25 to 50 deaths each year. The health hazards associated with landslides and mudflows include:
   a. Rapidly moving water and debris that can lead to trauma.
   b. Broken electrical, water, gas, and sewage lines that can result in injury or illness.
   c. Disrupted roadways and railways that can endanger motorists and disrupt transport and access to health care.
3. Some areas are more likely to experience landslides or mudflows.
   a. Areas where wildfires or human modification of the land have destroyed vegetation.
   b. Areas where landslides have occurred before.
   c. Steep slopes and areas at the bottom of slopes or canyons.
   d. Slopes that have been altered for construction of buildings and roads.
   e. Channels along a stream or river.
   f. Areas where surface runoff is directed.

C. Facility Action Plan.
1. Learn whether landslides or debris flows have occurred previously in your area by contacting local authorities, a county geologist, or the county planning department, state geological surveys or departments of natural resources, or university departments of geology.
2. Contact local authorities about emergency and evacuation plans.
3. During storms and rainfall, listen to the radio or watch TV for warnings about intense rainfall or for information and instructions from local officials.
4. If landslide or debris flow danger is imminent:
   a. Quickly move away from the path of the slide. Getting out of the path of a debris flow is your best protection.
   b. Move to the nearest high ground in a direction away from the path.
   c. If rocks and debris are approaching, run for the nearest shelter and take cover (if possible, under a desk, table, or other piece of sturdy furniture).
5. Consult a geotechnical expert (a registered professional engineer with soils engineering expertise) for advice on reducing additional landslide problems and risks. Local authorities should be able to tell you how to contact a geotechnical expert.
6. Locate and contact patients and staff as soon as possible post-event.

VIII. Volcanic eruptions.

A. Volcanoes.
1. Spew hot, dangerous gases, ash, lava, and rock that are powerfully destructive.
2. Ash is gritty, abrasive, sometimes corrosive, and always unpleasant.
   a. Small ash particles can abrade (scratch) the front of the eye.
   b. Ash particles may contain crystalline silica, a material that causes a respiratory disease called silicosis.
3. Volcanic eruptions may result in floods, landslides and mudslides, power outages, and wildfires.

B. Volcano facts.
1. The most common cause of death from a volcano is suffocation.
2. Volcanic eruptions can be accompanied by other natural hazards, including earthquakes, mudflows and flash floods, rockfalls and landslides, acid rain, fire, and (under special conditions) tsunamis.
3. Active volcanoes in the United States are found mainly in Hawaii, Alaska, and the Pacific Northwest. The danger area around a volcano covers approximately a 20-mile radius. However, some danger may exist 100 miles or more from a volcano.

4. Health concerns after a volcanic eruption.
   a. Infectious disease, respiratory illness, burns, injuries from falls, and vehicle accidents related to the slippery, hazy conditions caused by ash.
   b. When warnings are heeded, the chances of adverse health effects from a volcanic eruption are very low.
5. Volcanic gases.
   a. Most gases from a volcano quickly blow away. However, heavy gases such as carbon dioxide and hydrogen sulfide can collect in low-lying areas.
   b. Most common volcanic gas is water vapor, followed by carbon dioxide and sulfur dioxide. Sulfur dioxide can cause breathing problems in both healthy people and people with asthma and other respiratory problems.
   c. Other volcanic gases include hydrogen chloride, carbon monoxide, and hydrogen fluoride. Amounts of these gases vary widely from one volcanic eruption to the next.

C. Facility Action Plan.
1. Close all windows, doors, and fireplace or woodstove dampers.
2. Turn off all fans and heating and air conditioning systems.
3. Heed warnings and obey instructions from local authorities.
   a. Stay indoors until local health officials tell you it is safe to go outside.
   b. Listen to local news updates for information about air quality, drinking water, and roads.
4. Do not travel unless you have to.
   a. Driving in ash is hazardous to your health and your car.
   b. Driving will stir up more ash that can clog engines and stall vehicles.
5. Locate and contact patients and staff as soon as possible post-event.

IX. Tsunamis.

A. Tsunamis are a series of enormous waves created by an underwater disturbance such as an earthquake, landslide, volcanic eruption, or meteorite. A tsunami can move hundreds of miles per hour in the open ocean and smash into land with waves as high as 100 feet or more.

B. Tsunamis facts.
1. The topography of the coastline and the ocean floor will influence the size of the wave.
2. All tsunamis are potentially dangerous, even though they may not damage every coastline they strike. A tsunami can strike anywhere along most of the U.S. coastline. The most destructive tsunamis have occurred along the coasts of California, Oregon, Washington, Alaska, and Hawaii.
3. Earthquake-induced movement of the ocean floor most often generates tsunamis. If a major earthquake or landslide occurs close to shore, the first wave in a series could reach the beach in a few minutes, even before a warning is issued.
4. Drowning is the most common cause of death associated with a tsunami.
   a. Tsunami waves and the receding water are very destructive to structures.
   b. Other hazards include flooding, contamination of drinking water, and fires from gas lines or ruptured tanks.

C. Facility Action Plan.
1. If an earthquake occurs and you are in a coastal area, turn on your radio to learn if there is a tsunami warning.
2. Know the community's warning systems and disaster plans, including evacuation routes.
3. Know the height of your street above sea level and the distance of your street from the coast or other high-risk waters. Evacuation orders may be based on these numbers.
4. Turn off all utilities at the main power switch and close the main gas valve if evacuation appears necessary.
5. After the tsunami.
   a. Use caution when re-entering buildings or homes. Tsunami-driven floodwater may have damaged buildings where you least expect it.
   b. To avoid injury, wear protective clothing and be cautious when cleaning up.
   c. Patients and staff should have immunization records handy or be aware of last tetanus shot, in case of contamination from the flood waters.
   d. Account for all patients and staff.
6. Patient education and preparation.
   a. Patients should know where they will go if forced to evacuate.
   b. Periodically review procedures and drills for the emergency termination.
   c. If patients will have to miss a dialysis treatment, instruct them how to implement the emergency diet and fluid restriction plan.
   d. Patients need to tell shelter personnel about their special needs, such as diet and transportation to and from dialysis treatments.
7. Patients on in-center hemodialysis.
   a. If patients are dialyzing in the facility, the treatment should be stopped, using emergency protocols.
   b. Move patients into the designated safe area. Give physical assistance as needed.

8. Patients on home hemodialysis.
   a. Must be able to perform emergency disconnect procedures.
   b. The patient and partner should go to a safe area.
   c. Patients should register with local water and power company for priority reinstatement of services.
   d. If electrical power or water service is interrupted, patients must know how to contact the dialysis staff to make alternate dialysis arrangements.
9. Patients on peritoneal dialysis.
   a. An electrical outage will affect patients on continuous cycling peritoneal dialysis. These patients should possess the ability to perform manual exchanges during these times.
   b. If patients are unable to perform as many exchanges as ordered, they should have instructions to implement the emergency diet and fluid restrictions plan.
   c. Patients on peritoneal dialysis should have an emergency 5-day supply of antibiotics for potential peritonitis.
   d. Should be aware of emergency procedures to follow.
   e. When possible, they need to contact the facility to report their status.
   f. Should register with local water and power company for priority reinstatement of service.
   g. Know how to contact the dialysis staff to make alternate dialysis arrangements if there is a loss of power and/or water.
10. Patients receiving a transplant.
    a. Keep and carry a current list of their medications and keep a 2-week supply on hand.
    b. When possible, they need to contact the transplant center to report their status.
    c. Be aware of emergency procedures.
11. Patients with diabetes.
    a. Keep extra insulin and syringes.
    b. Keep extra batteries for glucometer.
    c. Patient should be aware of emergency procedures to follow.
12. All patients.
    a. Must move inland to higher ground immediately. A safe area should be 100 feet (30 meters) above sea level or as far as 2 miles (3 kilometers) inland, away from the coastline. Every foot inland or upward may make a difference.
    b. Keep and carry a current list of medications.
    c. Keep a 2-week supply of medication.
    d. Wear a medical information emblem.
    e. Have a battery-powered AM/FM radio and flashlight with extra batteries.
    f. Have a list of emergency phone numbers.
    g. Prepare themselves and their household the same ways as the general public.

SECTION C
Man-Made Disasters

I. Terrorism.

A. Threatens the public with widespread death and disease, fear, panic, and disruption to society, both psychologically and economically.

B. Terrorism is the use of force or violence against persons or property in violation of the criminal laws of the United States for purposes of intimidation, coercion, or ransom (FEMA, 2013).

C. Nurses need to comprehend their role in response to terrorist events, since they play a pivotal role in the assessment, diagnosis, and treatment of the victims of terrorism.

D. General safety guidelines.
   1. Be aware of your surroundings.
   2. Learn where emergency exits are located in the buildings you frequent.
   3. The facility should have portable battery-operated radio, flashlights with extra batteries, and a first-aid kit.

II. Bomb threat.

A. Potential bombing incidents constitute a serious threat to employees, patients, assets, operations, and facilities, whether the motive is found in extortion, assault, or an act of terror. This threat area has taken on relevance and is increasingly prevalent today for a number of reasons.
   1. Technology in the area of explosives and devices has advanced tremendously with the development and mass production of advanced electronics, plastics, and explosive materials.
   2. Materials necessary to construct a very powerful device are readily available from a wide variety of common sources.
   3. This information is increasingly and more readily available via "underground" publications and the Internet.

B. The options available to the well-planned attacker for effective placement of a device are numerous.

Delivery can be accomplished in any of a number of ways to include:
1. On the person of an employee, visitor, vendor, or maintenance person.
2. Within a box, purse, briefcase, or lunch box.
3. Via a commercial carrier, private delivery service, or the U.S. Postal Service.

C. Facility Action Plan.
1. In any size organization, employee involvement is the key to prevention.
   a. Provide employees with awareness training on the topic of bomb threats and extortion.
   b. Develop response policies and procedures.
   c. Consult with the local law enforcement and fire officials.
2. Bomb threats are usually received by telephone, the call is short in duration, and the caller usually refuses to answer questions.
3. The caller relies on the person taking the message being unable to determine the veracity of the threat statement. The caller will rely upon the person's inability to conduct an effective search of the facility in a very short period. If the caller can accomplish both of these objectives, the organization will be placed into a state of confusion and panic, which is most likely the caller's intent.
4. Is it a real threat situation, or not? Evacuate or not? Each of these decisions obviously carries a very serious question of safety. You will have to determine the validity of the threat with limited information on hand, and there will not be much time.
5. Proper preplanning and training are critical to this risk management process as you will have to:
   a. Quickly analyze the threat.
   b. Estimate the need for accurate response.
   c. Decide upon the most logical direction to take.
   d. Execute your plan.

III. Bioterrorism.

A. Bioterrorism is the intentional use of harmful biological substances or germs to cause widespread illness and fear. Smallpox, anthrax, botulism, nerve agents, ricin, and plague are examples of biological agents used in bioterrorism.

B. Facility Action Plan.
1. Check for instructions on local television, radio, and newspapers. In the event of a bioterrorism attack, it may take time to determine exactly what the illness is and how it should be treated.
2. Be prepared to discontinue treatments.

IV. Pandemics and influenza (flu).

A. Seasonal (or common) flu is a contagious respiratory illness caused by influenza viruses. Most people have some immunity, and a vaccine is available.

B. An influenza pandemic can occur when a non-human (novel) influenza virus gains the ability for efficient and sustained human-to-human transmission and then spreads globally. Influenza viruses that have the potential to cause a pandemic are referred to as "influenza viruses with pandemic potential" (CDC, 2014).

C. Avian flu, or bird flu, is caused by influenza viruses that occur naturally among wild birds.
1. The H5N1 variant is deadly to domestic fowl and can be transmitted from birds to humans.
2. In 2007, the FDA licensed the first vaccine in the United States for the prevention of H5N1 influenza. This inactivated influenza virus vaccine is for use in people 18 through 64 years of age who are at increased risk of exposure to the H5N1 influenza virus subtype contained in the vaccine.

D. Pandemic flu is a global outbreak of serious illness. Because there is little natural immunity, the disease can spread easily from person to person.
1. An influenza pandemic occurs when:
   a. A new influenza virus emerges for which there is little or no immunity in the human population.
   b. It begins to cause serious illness.
   c. It spreads easily person-to-person worldwide.
2. The federal government, states, communities, and industry are taking steps to prepare for and respond to an influenza pandemic outbreak.
3. A pandemic is likely to be a prolonged and widespread outbreak that could require temporary changes in many areas of society, such as schools, work, transportation, and other public services.
4. An informed and prepared public can take appropriate actions to decrease their risk during a pandemic (HHS, 2014).

E. Facility Action Plan.
1. Develop a preparedness plan as you would for other public health emergencies.
2. Review the ESRD checklist developed by the Department of Health and Human Services (DHHS) and the Centers for Disease Control (CDC) on http://www.pandemicflu.gov and http://www.cdc.gov
3. Participate and promote any public health efforts in your state and community.
4. Talk with your local public health officials; they can supply information about the signs and

symptoms of a specific disease outbreak.
5. Implement prevention and control actions recommended by your public health officials and providers.
6. Adopt practices that encourage sick employees to stay home.
7. Anticipate how to function with a significant portion of the workforce absent due to illness or caring for ill family members.
8. Wash hands frequently with soap and water.
9. Cover coughs and sneezes with tissues.
10. Stay informed about pandemic influenza and be prepared to respond.
11. Consult http://www.pandemicflu.gov frequently for updates on national and international information on pandemic influenza.

V. Chemical threat.

A. Chemical agents.
1. Poisonous vapors, aerosols, liquids, and solids that have a toxic effect of people, animals, and plants.
2. Some chemicals may be odorless and tasteless.
3. They can have an immediate (a few seconds to a few minutes) or delayed (2 to 48 hours) effect.

B. Chemical facts.
1. A chemical attack could come without warning.
2. Signs of a chemical release include people having difficulty breathing, eye irritation, loss of coordination, nausea, and burning sensation in nose and lungs.
3. Presence of dead birds and insects may indicate a chemical agent release.
4. Emergency Planning and Community Right to Know Act (EPCRA).
   a. Communities have a "right to know" about hazardous chemicals in the area.
   b. States are mandated to have an emergency response plan for chemical emergencies.
   c. The Occupational Safety and Health Administration's (OSHA) Hazardous Waste Operations and Emergency Response Standard mandates training for staff that may take care of patients exposed to toxic chemicals.

C. Facility Action Plan.
1. Ensure all employees have Hazard Communication (HAZCOM) Training.
2. The disaster supply kit should include a roll of duct tape, plastic, and scissors.
3. Identify an internal room without windows and on a high level as a safe room.
4. If instructed to remain in the facility:
   a. Close the doors and windows.
   b. Turn off all ventilation.
   c. Seal windows and doors with plastic.
5. Listen to the radio for further instruction by authorities.
6. After the attack, use extreme caution caring for those who have been exposed. Refer them to a hospital for further treatment.

VI. Workplace violence.

A. Any act in which a person is abused, threatened, intimidated, or assaulted in his/her place of employment is considered workplace violence.

B. Examples of workplace violence.
1. Threatening behavior – shaking fists, destroying property, throwing objects.
2. Verbal or written threats – any expression of intent to inflict harm.
3. Harassment – any unwelcome behavior that demeans, embarrasses, humiliates, annoys, alarms, or verbally abuses a person. This includes words, gestures, intimidation, or other inappropriate behavior.
4. Verbal abuse – swearing, insults, or condescending language.
5. Physical attacks – hitting, shoving, pushing or kicking.
6. Other examples – rumors, pranks, arguments, property damage, theft, anger-related incidents, arson, and murder.

C. Workplace violence facts.
1. According to OSHA (2013), 2 million American workers are victims of workplace violence each year.
2. Workplace violence is not limited to the traditional workplace. It can occur at off-site business related places (conferences) at social events related to work, even threatening phone calls.
3. Risk of violence can be greater at certain times of day, night, or year. For example: pay days, performance appraisals, late hours of the night, or early hours of the day.
4. Disruptive and hostile actions toward colleagues, hospital personnel, and patients or visitors can occur in the lives of nursing professionals. According to The Joint Commission (2010), these behaviors can take the form of:
   a. Hostile, angry, or aggressive confrontational voice or body language.
   b. Attacks (verbal or physical) that go beyond the bounds of fair professional conduct.
   c. Inappropriate expressions of anger such as destruction of property or throwing items.
   d. Abusive language or criticism directed in such a way as to ridicule, humiliate, intimidate, undermine, or belittle.

D. Facility Action Plan.
   1. Review any history of violence in the workplace.
   2. Determine any risk factors associated with workplace violence (AFSCME, 2012).
   3. Implement preventive measures such as:
      a. Position of lobby entrance.
      b. Position of furniture in offices.
      c. Installing physical barriers between the lobby and the clinic.
      d. Minimizing the number of entrances.
      e. Using code cards or keys for access to certain areas in the clinic.
      f. Installing alarm systems.
   4. Review *Decreasing Dialysis Patient Provider Conflict* toolbox from the Centers for Medicare and Medicaid Services (CMS, 2004): www.therenalnetwork.org/services/dpc.php
   5. Review OSHA workplace violence programs at http://www.osha.org (OSHA, 1989).
   6. Develop workplace policies and procedures to apply to management, employees, patients, vendors, and visitors.
      a. Provide clear examples of unacceptable behavior and their consequences.
      b. Outline the confidential process employees can use to report incidents.
      c. Outline the investigative process.
   7. Provide a confidential Employee Assistance Program (EAP) where employees can seek help.
   8. Implement additional strategies for bullying.
      a. Empower and educate their nursing colleagues to advocate for and role model respectful behavior.
      b. Provide information and education to other care providers on their role as supportive coworkers, and the negative effects of disruptive behavior on patient quality of care and patient and staff safety.
      c. Collaborate across organizational levels and disciplines to develop professional behavior programs that focus on providing support resources for staff.
      d. Set clear expectations for acceptable and unacceptable work behavior.
      e. Communicate and implement professional behavior policies, and act on reports of disruptive behavior and incivility according to planned policies procedures.
      f. Be alert and responsive to uncivil behaviors, including minor incidents of aggression or rudeness. Intervene early.
      g. Encourage your team to be supportive of each other.
      h. Listen and offer emotional support to staff and colleagues, especially during highly stressful times or after disruptive or aggressive incidents from patients or staff.
      i. Be accountable to colleagues and other staff when addressing disruptive behavior and incivility from others or oneself (Yragui et al., 2013).

Note: More information can be found online. See Table 4.3 for additional resources.

SECTION D
Disaster Drills

I. Effective drills.

A. Practice and train in emergency response.
   1. Use meaningful and varied drills that involve different scenarios likely to be experienced.
   2. The amount of time needed to evacuate the facility may depend on the type of disaster.

B. To ensure competency during an emergency or disaster, there should be regularly scheduled response drills.
   1. Rehearse roles and tasks.
   2. Identify and use resources.
   3. Pose scenarios to the staff:
      a. How long would it take to evacuate the facility?
      b. Does the time to evacuate differ from shift to shift?
      c. How many patients will need assistance for emergency termination?
      d. How many patients need assistance to evacuate the facility?
      e. What if the designated safe area is compromised?

II. Incident Command System (ICS).

A. In the 1970s, ICS was developed for first responders, and later adapted for hospital use (National Incident Management System [NIMS], 2004).

B. ICS is used throughout the United States and internationally by police and fire departments, health providers, and other organizations.

C. ICS is familiar to emergency responders who understand communications and actions taken using this system.

D. ICS is geared toward making people self-sufficient in an emergency, instead of relying on outside emergency responders for decision making.
   1. The ICS is a widely applicable management system

Table 4.3

Online Resources

Association	Website
American Association of Kidney Patients (AAKP)	https://www.aakp.org
American Hospital Association (AHA)	http://www.hospitalconnect.com
American Kidney Fund (AKF)	http://www.kidneyfund.org
American Nephrology Nurses' Association (ANNA)	http://www.annanurse.org
American Nurses Association (ANA)	http://www.nursingworld.org
American Red Cross	http://www.redcross.org
Association of Organ Procurement Organizations (AOPO)	http://www.aopo.org
Citizen Corps	http://www.citizencorps.gov
Centers for Disease Control and Prevention (CDC)	http://www.cdc.gov http://www.pandemicflu.gov
Center for Medicare and Medicaid Services (CMS)	http://cms.hhs.gov
Federal Emergency Management Agency (FEMA)	http://www.fema.gov
Forum of ESRD Networks	http://www.esrdnetworks.org
Kidney Community Emergency Response Coalition (KCERC)	http://www.KCERCoalition.com 1-888-33KIDNEY (1-888-335-4363)
National Council of State Boards of Nursing (NCSBN)	http://www.ncsbn.org
National Weather Service (NWS)	http://www.weather.gov
National Hurricane Center (NHC)	http://www.nhc.noaa.gov
National Kidney Foundation (NKF)	http://www.kidney.org
The Weather Channel	http://www.weather.com
United States Geological Survey (USGS)	http://pubs.usgs.gov http://water.usgs.gov/osw/
United States Environmental Protection Agency (EPA)	http://www.epa.gov

designed to enable effective, efficient incident management by integrating a combination of facilities, equipment, personnel, procedures, and communications operating within a common organizational structure.

2. It represents organizational "best practices" and, as an element of the Command and Management Component of NIMS, has become the standard for emergency management across the country.
3. Designers recognized early that ICS must be interdisciplinary and organizationally flexible to:
   a. Meet the needs of incidents of any kind or size.
   b. Allow personnel from a variety of agencies to work together in a common management structure.
   c. Provide logistical and administrative support to staff.
   d. Avoid duplication of efforts.

III. Training of staff. (Table 4.4 details necessary core competencies for nephrology nurses in emergency response.)

A. Step 1: Train staff for implementation of emergency drills using the Incident Command System (ICS).
   1. Review the organizational structure of ICS.
   2. Explain differences in terminology (see Table 4.5 for ICS terminology).
   3. Review role and responsibilities of staff during drill.

Table 4.4

Core Competencies for Nephrology Nursing Emergency Response

Standard	Objectives	Competencies	Strategies
Assessment	The nephrology registered nurse collects comprehensive data pertinent to the healthcare consumer's health and/or situation.	Assess possible threat. Identify barriers to education regarding emergency response plan. Make appropriate decisions based on analysis of gathered information. Take appropriate action based on assessed risks.	Receipt of alerts from EMS, EOC, National weather service, departments of public safety and public health. Review Emergency response plan. Physical/psychological factors: dementia, impaired mobility, advanced age, comorbidities, nonadherence.
Planning	The nephrology registered nurse develops a plan that prescribes strategies and alternatives to attain expected outcomes.	Develop an individualized plan for self and healthcare consumer. Integrates current scientific evidence, trends, and research. Develop and implement plans and gain concurrence of affected agencies and/or the public. Development of crisis standards.	If enough warning, dialyze patients prior to the event. Give patient disaster packet with individualized information. Ensure adequate supplies for patient and facility. Transfer patients (as needed) to shelters and/or areas outside of disaster zone.
Implementation	The nephrology registered nurse implements the identified plan.	Partners with Network, EOC. Communication styles.	Influence, guide, and direct assigned personnel to accomplish objectives and desired outcomes. Use suitable communication techniques to share relevant information with patients and personnel on a timely basis.
Coordination of Care	The nephrology registered nurse coordinates care delivery.	Demonstrates ability to manage care and resources. Assists patients to identify options. Proficient in communication during emergency situations. Documents care.	Coordinates patient tracking system with Networks, KCER, and EOC. Transportation. Complications. Ensure relevant information is exchanged during briefings. Ensure documentation is complete and disposition is appropriate.
Evaluation	The nephrology registered nurse evaluates progress toward attainment of outcomes.	Evaluate disaster situation. Evaluate drills. Reevaluate. Document.	Assess impact on patients. Include a psychological needs assessment. Disseminates results of drills/actual responses. Evaluate actions to complete assignments safely and meet identified objectives. Ensure documentation is complete.

Table 4.5

The Incident Command System

Section	Description
Incident Command Section	The command function is directed by the Incident Commander, who is the person in charge at the incident, and who must be fully qualified to manage the response. Major responsibilities for the Incident Commander include: • Protecting life and property. • Controlling personnel and equipment resources. • Maintaining accountability for responder and public safety, as well as for task accomplishment. • Establishing and maintaining an effective liaison with outside agencies and organizations, including the EOC, when it is activated. • Coordinating overall emergency activities. • Coordinating the activities of outside agencies. • Authorizing the release of information to the media. • Keeping track of costs. Qualifications: assertive, decisive, objective, calm, quick thinking. When expansion is required, the Incident Commander will establish other Command Staff positions: Information Officer, Safety Officer, Liaison Officer. • Information Officer handles all media inquiries and coordinates the release of information to the media with the Public Affairs Officer at the EOC • Safety Officer monitors safety conditions and develops measures for ensuring the safety of assigned personnel and patients. • Liaison Officer is the on-scene contact for other agencies assigned to the incident.
Planning Section	In smaller events, the Incident Commander is responsible for planning, but when the incident is of larger scale, the Incident Commander establishes the Planning Section. The Planning Section's function includes the collection, evaluation, dissemination, and use of information about the development of the incident and status of resources.
Operations Section	The Operations Section is responsible for carrying out the response activities. The Operations Section Chief reports to the Incident Commander and determines the required resources and organizational structure. The Operations Section Chief's main responsibilities are to: • Direct and coordinate all operations, ensuring the safety of Operations Section personnel. • Assist the Incident Commander in developing response goals and objectives for the incident. • Implement an Incident Action Plan. • Request (or release) resources through the Incident Commander. • Keep the Incident Commander informed of situation and resource status within operations.
Logistics Section	The Logistics Section is responsible for providing facilities, services, and materials, including personnel to operate the requested equipment for the incident.
Finance Section	The Finance/Administration Section is critical for tracking incident costs and reimbursement accounting. Unless costs and financial operations are carefully recorded and justified, reimbursement of costs is difficult, if not impossible.

4. Train on skills needed for each scenario (e.g., use of fire extinguishers during fire drill).

B. Step 2: Get the facility ready for an emergency drill using ICS. Functional responsibilities to be covered in an ICS drill include:
   1. Healthcare: triaging and treating.
   2. Logistics and operations: assessing damages and casualties, providing support to healthcare teams, and managing security of building and records.
   3. Communications: directing all post-emergency communications, including those with media.
   4. Documentation: recording information about the incident, causalities, damage, and actions taken in response to the incident.
   5. Dispatch: Assembling and dispatching persons to respond to needs as directed.

C. Step 3: Plan, conduct, and evaluate drills each quarter.
   1. Divide staff into teams.
   2. Identify Incident Commander. Rotate so all staff have experience with leading the drill.
   3. Conduct the drill. Drills should reflect each possible scenario that may affect the facility.
   4. Provide support and supplies.
   5. Evaluate and assess.

IV. Altered standards of care.

A. The Standards of Professional Performance describe a competent level of behavior in the professional role, including activities related to quality of practice, education, professional practice evaluation, collegiality, collaboration, ethics, research, resource utilization, and leadership.

B. The Centers for Disease Control and Prevention (CDC), the Public Health Department, and the American Nurses Association (ANA) are developing crisis standards to be followed during a large-scale disaster.

C. The patient with kidney disease is vulnerable to decreasing healthcare resources not only in a large-scale disaster, but in the current healthcare environment constrained by budget shortfalls.

D. The most critical standards for nurses.
   1. Maximizing staff and patient safety.
   2. Maintaining airway and breathing, circulation, and control of blood loss.
   3. Maintaining or establishing infection control practices.

V. Resources for training.

A. National Incident Management System (NIMS).
   1. All sectors of health care are required to use a common incident management/response system. The NIMS plan is an evolving document, and can be readily accessed through the Federal Emergency Management Agency (FEMA) Emergency Management Institute website (FEMA, 2014) http://www.training.fema.gov/IS/
   2. Nurses will need to be thoroughly versed in NIMS and the incident command system (ICS) and be personally and professionally prepared to respond to any type of emergency event.

B. Centers for Disease Control (CDC).
   1. Emergency response begins at the local level. CDC prepares local and state public health departments by providing funding and technical assistance to strengthen their abilities to respond to all types of emergencies and build more resilient communities.
   2. When local and state resources become overwhelmed, CDC responds and supports national, state, and local partners to save lives and reduce suffering. This includes providing scientific and logistic expertise, and deploying personnel and critical medical assets to the site of an emergency.
   3. CDC also helps these partners recover and restore public health functions after the initial response.

C. Clinicians Outreach and Communications Activity (COCA).
   1. The CDC Emergency Communication System's Clinician Communication Team manages the Clinician Outreach Communication Activity (COCA) to ensure that clinicians have the up-to-date information they need.
   2. COCA is designed to provide two-way communication between clinicians and the CDC about emerging health threats, such as pandemics, natural disasters, and terrorism.

D. National Institute for Occupational Safety and Health (NIOSH).
   1. The National Institute for Occupational Safety and Health (NIOSH) is the U.S. federal agency that conducts research and makes recommendations to prevent worker injury and illness.
   2. NIOSH is part of the U.S. Centers for Disease Control and Prevention, in the U.S. Department of Health and Human Services.
   3. NIOSH provides the only dedicated federal investment for research needed to prevent the societal cost of work-related fatalities, injuries, and illnesses in the United States.
   4. NIOSH works to promote a healthy, safe, and capable workforce.

E. American Red Cross.
   1. The Red Cross responds to approximately 70,000 disasters in the United States every year, ranging from home fires that affect a single family to hurricanes that affect tens of thousands, to earthquakes that impact millions.
   2. In these events, the Red Cross provides shelter, food, health services, and mental health services to help families and entire communities get back on their feet.

F. Federal Emergency Management Agency (FEMA).
   1. The Federal Emergency Management Agency coordinates the federal government's role in preparing for, preventing, mitigating the effects of, responding to, and recovering from all domestic disasters, whether natural or man-made, including acts of terror.
   2. To take a course at Emergency Management Institute (EMI), applicants must meet the selection criteria and prerequisites specified for each course.
   3. EMI courses are generally limited to U.S. residents. However, each year a limited number of international participants are accommodated in Emergency Management Institute courses.

G. Kidney Community Emergency Response Coalition (KCER).
   1. KCER Coalition provides technical assistance to ESRD Networks, Medicare organizations, and other groups to ensure timely and efficient disaster preparedness, response, and recovery for the kidney community.
   2. KCER Coalition strives to provide disaster preparedness resources to save lives, improve

outcomes, empower patients and families, educate healthcare workers, build partnerships with stakeholders, promote readiness in the community, and support the ESRD Network Program.

3. Response teams. Currently eight response teams focus on these eight areas of preparedness and response activities:
   a. Training and education.
      (1) Development of a training program to enhance the kidney community, to include the patients and providers and response capabilities.
      (2) Development of training materials to include exercises and drills to test the ability to implement the Plan through annual regional or national exercises.
   b. Coordination of staff and volunteers: database of nurses, dialysis technicians, social workers, and dietitians.
   c. Physician: tools to assist physicians prepare and respond to a disaster.
   d. Executive: leaders of all the committees meet to discuss the accomplishments and project vision for the future to strengthen the ESRD community.
   e. Facility operations: facilitate cooperative planning among the wide variety of dialysis facilities, ESRD Networks, and community disaster planners; assist with facility preparation, response, and recovery efforts.
   f. Communications: Kidney Care Emergency website and toll-free numbers.
   g. Federal response: education that was distributed to federal, state, and local emergency responders regarding the needs of individuals with kidney failure.
   h. Pandemic and infectious disease: plans in the event of a pandemic flu or other infectious disease.

References

American Federation of State, County Municipal Employees. (2012). (AFSCME). *Workplace violence fact sheet.* Retrieved from http://www.afscme.org/news/publications/workplace-health-and-safety/fact-sheets

American Nurses Association (ANA). (2002). *Position statement on registered nurses' rights and responsibilities related to work release during a disaster.* Retrieved from http://nursingworld.org/responsibilitiesdisasterps

Centers for Disease Control and Prevention (CDC). (2014). Updated preparedness and response framework for influenza pandemics. *Morbidity and Mortality Weekly Report, 63*(RR06), 1-9.

Centers for Medicare and Medicaid Services (CMS). (2005). *Decreasing dialysis patient provider conflict.* CMS contract #500-03-NW14 with the ESRD Network of Texas, Inc. Retrieved from http://www.therenalnetwork.org/services/dpc.php

Centers for Medicare and Medicaid Services (CMS). (2008). *Disaster preparedness: A guide for chronic dialysis facilities* (2nd ed). Publication number HHSM-500-2010-NW007C. Retrieved from http://www.kcercoalition.com

Counts, C. (2001). Disaster preparedness: Is your unit ready? *Nephrology Nursing Journal,* 28(5), 491-499.

Federal Emergency Management Agency. (2014). *Emergency Management Institute. FEMA Independent study program: IS-100 Introduction to Incident Command System (ICS/NIMS).* Retrieved from http://www.training.fema.gov/IS/

Federal Emergency Management Agency (FEMA). (2014). *Main page.* http://www.ready.gov

Kopp, J.B., Ball, L.K., Cohen, A., Kenney, R.J., Lempert, K.D., Miller, P.E., … Yelton, S.A. (2007). Kidney patient care in disasters: Lessons from the hurricanes and earthquake of 2005. *Clinical Journal of the American Society of Nephrology, 2*(4), 814-824.

Lettieri, C. (2006). Disaster medicine: Understanding the threat and minimizing the effects. *Medscape Emergency Medicine, 1*(1).

National Child Traumatic Stress Network (NCTSN) and National Center for PTSD. (2007). *Psychological first aid: Field operations guide* (2nd ed.). Retrieved from http://www.nctsn.org/content/psychological-first-aid

National Hurricane Center (n.d.) *Hurricane preparedness.* Retrieved from http://www.nhc.noaa.gov

Occupational Safety and Health Administration (OSHA). (1989). *Safety and health management program guidelines.* Retrieved from http://www.osha.org

Qureshi, K., Gershon, R., Gebbie, E., Straub, T., & Morse, S. (2005). Healthcare workers ability and willingness to report to duty during a catastrophic disaster. *Journal of Urban Health, 82*(3), 378-88.

The Joint Commission. (2010, June 3). Preventing violence in the health care setting. *Sentinel Event Alert,* Issue 45. Retrieved from http://www.jointcommission.org/sentinel_event_alert_issue_45_preventing_violence_in_the_health_care_setting_/

United States Department of Health and Human Services (HHS). (2014). FLU.GOV: *Pandemic flu.* Retrieved from http://www.flu.gov/pandemic/about

United States Geological Survey (USGS). (2006). *Flood hazards – A national threat.* Retrieved from http://pubs.er.usgs.gov/publication/fs20063026

Yragui, N., Silverstein, B., & Johnson, W. (2013). Stopping the pain: The role of nurse leaders in providing organizational resources to reduce disruptive behavior. *American Nurse Today, 8*(10). Retrieved from http://www.americannursetoday.com

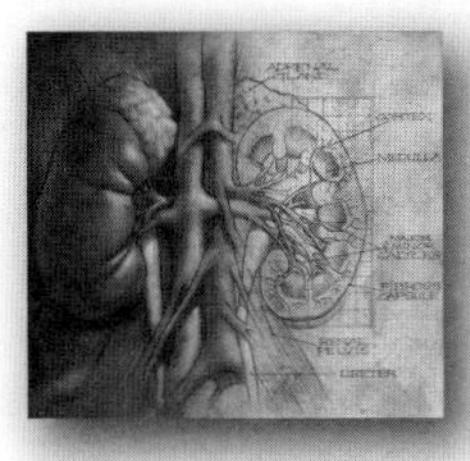

Self-Assessment Questions for Module 1

These questions apply to all chapters in Module 1 and can be used for self-testing. They are not considered part of the official CNE process.

Chapter 1

1. The Nursing Licensure Compact (NLC) is a method to
   a. allow a licensed nurse to practice in all states of the United States.
   b. extend to nurses the ability to practice in states that participate in the NLC.
   c. standardize the nursing licensure requirements in all states.
   d. decrease the responsibilities of individual State Boards of Nursing.

2. The ethical principle that supported the passage of the law that allowed Medicare coverage of dialysis and kidney transplantation was
   a. beneficence.
   b. utilitarianism.
   c. fidelity.
   d. veracity.

3. The best questions to assist in predicting how an interviewee will manage in a position are those that
   a. focus on personal characteristics.
   b. ask about the types of jobs held previously.
   c. query about his family and plans for the future.
   d. require answering how situations should be managed.

4. Behaviors that help create a healthy work setting include
   a. being respectful, setting limits on bullying, and exclusive employee groups.
   b. using common courtesies, being inclusive, acculturation of new graduates.
   c. inclusivity, limited discussion of problems, and discouraging cliques.
   d. zero tolerance for bullying, exclusivity, and centralized decision making.

5. Preparing for a CMS visit requires that
   a. one person must be responsible for all the preparation.
   b. identify a person to assure that policies are rewritten.
   c. familiarity with the Medicare Standards and Conditions related to dialysis.
   d. developing tracking tools for each dialysis unit in the system.

Chapter 2

6. Which of the following underlying principles influences nursing practice? The need to
   a. provide age-appropriate, culturally and ethnically sensitive care.
   b. realize that all patients may not need continuity of care.
   c. demonstrate that care collaboration ends upon admission to an acute care setting.
   d. educate patients only when requested.

7. Which of the following is correct regarding the NKF-KDOQI guidelines?
   a. The KDOQI are not standards of care.
   b. The KDOQI guidelines are based on expert opinion.
   c. The KDOQI guidelines are developed by nurses serving on work groups.
   d. The KDOQI guidelines improve outcomes for individuals with acute kidney injury.

8. Depression is considered to be
   a. a predictor of morbidity.
   b. a predictor of loss vascular access.
   c. a key quality of life indicator.
   d. difficult to assess.

9. A critical assessment and evaluation of research studies focusing on a specific clinical question through the use of identified methods to limit bias define
   a. a systematic review.
   b. qualitative data.
   c. quantitative data.
   d. a randomized control trial.

10. Which of the following is an extensive national database that collects, analyzes, and distributes information about end-stage renal disease in the United States?
    a. USRDS
    b. DOPPS
    c. UNOS
    d. KDOQI

11. According to CROWNWeb data, the number of dialysis and transplant patients treated for ESRD increases by how much each year?
    a. 1%
    b. 2–3%
    c. 5%
    d. 10%
12. What piece of legislation prohibited the purchase of human organs?
    a. National Organ Transplant Act of 1984.
    b. Uniform Anatomical Gift Act of 1968.
    c. The first OPTN contract in 1986.
    d. Guidelines written by the South-Eastern. Procurement Foundation in 1975.
13. Data reports published by UNOS include which of the following types of information?
    a. National.
    b. State.
    c. Transplant-center specific.
    d. All of the above.

Chapter 3

14. When introducing legislation, which of the following is true?
    a. Proposed bills must be introduced in the House and Senate.
    b. Thousands of bills are introduced and enacted every congressional session.
    c. Ideas can come from any citizen.
    d. If a bill is not acted upon over the course of a year, it dies at the end of the session.
15. Nurses should recognize their role in advocacy for all of the following reasons EXCEPT:
    a. The ability to practice as a nurse is impacted by legislation and regulation.
    b. Members of Congress are knowledgeable about health care.
    c. The perception of nurses is that they are honest and ethical.
    d. Nurses are knowledgeable about the needs of patients.
16. If the president vetos a bill, what percent of Congress can override the presidential veto?
    a. One half.
    b. Two thirds.
    c. Three quarters.
17. Which of the following is NOT TRUE about Nurse Practice Acts:
    a. All states have a Nurse Practice Act.
    b. They are governed by the states.
    c. They define the functions of nursing.
    d. They set standards for licensure.
18. Which of the following is NOT TRUE about the development of the federal budget?
    a. Discretionary programs must be funded and renewed each year or defined interval.
    b. May include changes to mandatory or entitlement programs.
    c. Must include changes to the tax code.
19. State government is responsible for all of the following EXCEPT:
    a. ownership of property.
    b. implementation of welfare and other benefit programs.
    c. maintenance of a justice system.
    d. implementation of tax laws.
    e. education of inhabitants.
20. Which of the following is/are true about being politically active?
    a. Register and vote in elections.
    b. Learning about state and federal issues.
    c. Work with state board of nursing regarding changes to practice.
    d. Volunteer on an election campaign.
    e. Educating elected officials.
    f. a, b, d, e.
    g. b, c, d, e.
    h. All the above.
21. Which of the following impact healthcare policy?
    a. Nursing shortage.
    b. Aging nursing workforce.
    c. Patient safety.
    d. Economic environment.
    e. Safe work practices.
    f. a, b, c, e.
    g. All the above.
22. Educating elected officials includes all the following EXCEPT:
    a. Do your homework on an issue.
    b. Have a clear and concise message.
    c. Provide all the information you are able to obtain.
    d. Offer assistance to your representative.

True or False

23. Authorization of a bill ensures the provision of funds for the bill have been approved.
24. Bills may be referred to more than one committee and may be split into parts and sent to different committees.
25. All states are composed of two chambers: a Senate and General Assembly or House of Representatives.

Chapter 4

26. An example of a natural disaster is
    a. war.
    b. bioterrorism.
    c. nuclear accident.
    d. volcanic eruption.

27. The key to effective disaster management is
    a. risk assessment.
    b. post-disaster mitigation.
    c. pre-disaster planning and preparation.
    d. having all administrative personnel on the planning committee.

28. What action should you NOT take during an earthquake?
    a. Face away from the windows.
    b. Start immediate termination procedures.
    c. Keep machine wheels locked at all times.
    d. Have patients protect their head and access.

29. Tornados generally last
    a. 10 minutes.
    b. 20 minutes.
    c. 1 hour.
    d. 2 hours or more.

30. The leading cause of death in a winter storm is
    a. heart attack.
    b. hypothermia.
    c. asphyxiation.
    d. ice- and snow-related automobile accidents.

31. Bioterrorism includes all but the following:
    a. Ricin.
    b. Anthrax.
    c. Asian flu.
    d. Small pox.

32. Which of the following questions is/are appropriate to ask to determine if the facility is ready to respond to a disaster?
    a. Do you perform disaster drills?
    b. Do you have a written disaster plan?
    c. How do you communicate to your staff and patients when the facility is closed?
    d. All of the above

33. The pre-event phase is focused on
    a. implementation of the plan.
    b. anticipation, planning, and training.
    c. minimizing the negative impact of the event.
    d. risk assessment, communication, and mitigation.

34. Prior to using a generator as part of the disaster plan, what must be assessed?
    a. Maintenance log.
    b. Size of generator needed.
    c. Fuel and fuel storage availability.
    d. All of the above.

35. The most common health concern after a volcanic eruption is
    a. heavy gases.
    b. infectious disease.
    c. respiratory illness.
    d. injuries from falls.

Answer Key

Chapter 1
1. b
2. a
3. d
4. b
5. c

Chapter 2

6. a
7. a
8. c
9. a
10. a
11. b
12. a
13. d

Chapter 3

14. c
15. b
16. b
17. a
18. c
19. d
20. h
21. g
22. c
23. False
24. True
25. False

Chapter 4

26. d
27. c
28. b
29. a
30. d
31. c
32. d
33. b
34. d
35. c

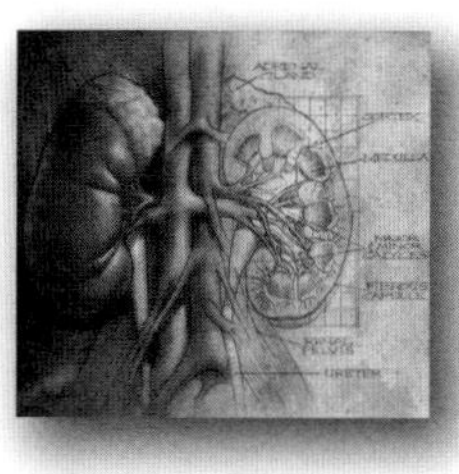

Index for Module 1

Page numbers followed by **f** indicate figures.
Page numbers followed by **t** indicate tables

G

H

I

J

K

Q

R

S

T

U

V

W